Student's G
Veterinary Medical
Terminology

Phillip E. Cochran, MS, DVM
Portland Community College
Rock Creek Campus
17705 NW Springville Road
PO Box 19000
Portland, Oregon 97219-0990

Technical Editor: Joann Colville, DVM
Book Editor: Paul W. Pratt, VMD
Production Manager: Elisabeth S. Stein

American Veterinary Publications, Inc.
5782 Thornwood Drive
Goleta, California 93117

While every effort has been made to en-
sure the accuracy of information contained herein, the publisher and author
are not legally responsible for errors or
omissions.

Library of Congress Card Number: 90-85893

ISBN 0-939674-31-9

Printed in the United States of America

Preface

This guide was written to help students of veterinary technology (animal health technology), veterinary science or veterinary medicine understand the construction, meaning and pronunciation of terms used in veterinary medicine. The vocabulary of the veterinary profession differs significantly from that of human medicine, such that texts and courses offered in human medical terminology do not adequately fulfill the instructional needs of students of veterinary science.

Instead of presenting a long list of medical words for memorization, this guide presents the proper rules of word construction and word analysis, enabling the student to construct or define medical words based on an understanding of their component parts.

This guide assumes no extensive knowledge of anatomy or physiology, other than that learned in college or high school biology classes. A medical dictionary should be purchased to aid in mastery of medical terminology.

This book has been designed in the form of a programmed guide so as to provide information in a sequential learning order. It can be used with an instructor in a classroom situation, or as a self-study guide for students interested in learning this subject through independent study.

An instructor may choose to deviate from the order in which these lessons are listed. This deviation might be necessary and appropriate if this book is used in a course taught concurrently with a course in anatomy or physiology. In this situation, Lesson 8, which presents directional and positional terms, might be taught between the first and second lessons. This would be necessary because dissection manuals use these directional and positional terms in their descriptions for dissecting animals.

Each definition in the glossary (Appendix 2) was derived from the sources listed in the Bibliography (Appendix 3). Most of the pronunciations were derived from *Dorland's Illustrated Medical Dictionary*.

In this guide, accented syllables are printed in CAPITAL LETTERS. Syllables not accented are printed in small letters. In multisyllabic words with primary and secondary accents, the syllable with the primary (greater) accent is printed in **BOLDFACED CAPITAL LETTERS**, while the syllable with the secondary (lesser) accent is printed in CAPITAL LETTERS only. Unaccented syllables are printed in small letters. Words of one syllable are printed in small letters. Multisyllabic words in which all syllables receive equal stress are printed in small letters.

Phillip E. Cochran, MS, DVM

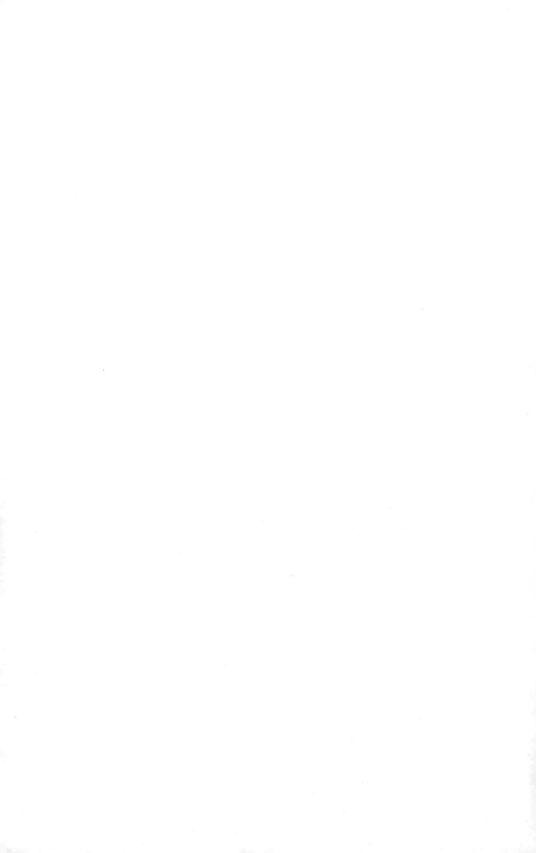

Contents

Lesson 1

Use of Nouns, Adjectives and Verbs

Nouns vs Adjectives

Nouns are words naming or denoting a person, place, thing, action or quality. Dog, blood, pain and joint are nouns. *Adjectives* are words used to limit or qualify a noun; they describe or modify (change the meaning of) nouns and make them more precise. Big, red and sore are adjectives.

Example: big dog

red hair

joint pain

sore joint

Note that the word *joint* is used as both an adjective and a noun. In the third example, it is an adjective that qualifies or specifies the location of the pain. In the fourth example, it is a noun denoting the anatomic part that is sore.

Note: Throughout this book, syllables with a primary (greater) accent are printed in **BOLDFACED CAPITAL LETTERS**, while syllables with a secondary (lesser) accent are printed in CAPITAL LETTERS only. Unaccented syllables are printed in small letters.

1

The spelling of a word can distinguish noun and adjective forms when the words are phonetically similar in pronunciation.

Examples: **MU**cous (adjective), as in mucous membranes

MUcus (noun), as in production of mucus

EStrous (adjective), as in estrous cycle

EStrus (noun), as in being in estrus

Note that the adjective forms of the above words end with the letters "-ous." Numerous other word endings designate the adjective form. In medical terminology this often occurs when a combining form (to be discussed later in this lesson) is joined with the word ending for adjectives. This forms an adjective that is used similarly to the adjective of the word *joint.* That is, it specifies a location. Common word endings that denote an adjective are the following:

-ac, as in **CAR**diac (pertaining to the heart)

-ar, as in **MUS**cular (pertaining to the muscles)

-al, as in **FEM**oral (pertaining to the femur)

-ic, as in trau**MA**tic (pertaining to trauma)

-ous, as in **MU**cous (pertaining to mucus-
            producing tissues)

When adjectives are defined, the definitions often start with the phrase "pertaining to" or "concerning the." However, if the definition is to indicate a motion, direction or location, it usually does not use the phrase "pertaining to," as in the following examples:

SUBcu**TA**neous, meaning under the skin

PERi**A**nal, meaning around the anus

PERi**CAR**dial, meaning around the heart

Two exceptions to the above rule are the endings "-ic" and "-al." They are also used to form a number of nouns, especially pharmacologic nouns, such as antibiotic, cathartic, anti-diarrheal and biological.

Verbs

Verbs are words showing action or a state of being. They are mainly used in their infinitive form, which means "to ----." The following are examples of verbs:

> in**HALE**, meaning to breathe in
>
> ex**HALE**, meaning to breathe out

Adjectives and Nouns as Applied to Different Species

The nouns listed below indicate names for common domestic species. the adjectives are the Latin derivation of the word in adjective form, such as *canine* from the Latin word *canis*.

Noun	Adjective
dog	**CA**nine
cat	**FE**line
horse	**E**quine
ox (cattle)	**BO**vine
sheep	**O**vine
goat	**CA**prine
pig	**POR**cine
bird	**A**vian
mouse, rat	**MU**rine
parrot	**PSIT**tacine

The use of the above words is illustrated in the following examples:

SURgery of the dog

Canine surgery

It is quite common to speak of a dog as a canine or list "canine" as the species on veterinary records. This is appropriate, as "canine" can be used as an adjective or a noun.

Word Drill A

In the blank space provided, convert the phrase using the noun to a phrase using the corresponding adjective form (numbers 1-5), and *vice versa* (numbers 6-10). The correct answers are listed in Appendix 1.

Example:

Use of the Noun	Use of the Adjective
Pa**THOL**ogy of birds	Avian pathology
1. Surgery of horses	1.
2. **MED**icine of dogs	2.
3. In**FEC**tious a**NE**mia of cats	3.
4. **IN**flu**EN**za of pigs	4.
5. **LEP**tospi**RO**sis of sheep	5.
6.	6. Murine pneumonia
7.	7. Bovine **DI**ar**RHE**a
8.	8. Caprine mas**TI**tis
9.	9. Psittacine beak and feather disease
10.	10. Canine estrous cycle

Introduction to Medical Words

Definitions

Prefix: A syllable, group of syllables or word united with or joined to the beginning of another word to alter its meaning or create a new word. *Example:* Bi-: meaning 2 or twice.

Root Word: The part of the word consisting of a syllable, group of syllables or word that is the basis (or word base) for the meaning of the word. *Example:* **CAR**di-: the root word (or "root") referring to the heart.

Combining Form: A word or root word that may or may not use the connecting vowel "o" when used as an element in word formation. That is, it is the combination of the root word and the combining vowel. It is generally written as "root word"/o. *Example:* **CAR**di/o: the combining form for the heart, where "cardi" is the root word and "/o" is the combining vowel (see below).

Combining Vowel: The vowel, usually an "o," used to connect a word or root word to the appropriate suffix.

Suffix: A syllable, group of syllables or word added at the end of a word to change its meaning, give it grammatic function or form a new word. *Example:* -logy: the study of (as in cardiology).

Compound Word: Two or more words combined to make a new word. *Example:* **HORSE**fly: the words horse and fly combined.

Rules for Word Construction

Use of the Prefix

The prefix is attached to the beginning of the root word to form an altered or new word.

Prefix	Root Word	Combination	Definition
de-	horn	dehorn	To remove the horns
semi-	permeable	semipermeable	Allowing only certain elements or liquids to pass through a membrane
pre-	operative	preoperative	Before surgery

Use of the Suffix

The suffix is attached to the end of the root word to form an altered or new word.

Root Word	Suffix	Combination	Definition
TONsil	-itis	**TON**sil**I**tis	Inflammation of the tonsils
THYroid	-ectomy	**THY**roid**EC**tomy	Removal of the thyroid gland
al**BU**min	-uria	al**BU**mi**NU**ria	Albumin in the urine

Compound Word

Two words are joined together to form a new word.

Word 1	Word 2	Combination	Definition
heart	beat	**HEART**beat	Pulsation of the heart
blood	worms	**BLOOD**worms	Worms (nematodes) that get into a main artery of the intestines in horses
lock	jaw	**LOCK**jaw	Colloquial term for tetanus

Combining Forms

Certain rules are peculiar to use of combining forms and the combining vowel "o." These are as follows:

- *If the suffix begins with a consonant, use the combining vowel "o" with the root word (the combining form) to which the suffix will be added. Example:* Cardi/o (combining form for heart) plus -megaly (enlargement of) to form the combined form CARdiomegaly, which means enlargement of the heart.
- *Do not use the combining vowel "o" when the suffix begins with a vowel. Example:* Hepat/o (combining form for liver) plus -osis (a condition, disease or morbid process) to form the combined form HEPaTOsis, which means a disease of the liver.
- *If the suffix begins with the same vowel that the combining form ends with (minus the combining vowel "o"), do not repeat the vowel twice when forming the new word. Example:* Cardi/o minus the "o" leaves Cardi-. Adding -itis (inflammation of) forms carditis, which means inflammation of the heart. As the rule states, the combined form, carditis, has only 1 "i."

Combining Form	Suffix	Combination	Definition
cardi/o	-logy	CARdiOLogy	Study of heart function and disease
mast/o	-itis	masTItis	Inflammation of the mammary glands
BRONch/o	-spasm	BRONchospasm	Spasm of the bronchus

Using Only the Prefix and Suffix To Form Words

In this situation, no root word is used. The prefix is added directly to the suffix.

Prefix	Suffix	Combination	Definition
dys-	-uria	dysUria	Trouble urinating
POLy-	-phagia	POLyPHAGia	Eating excessively
an-	-emia	aNEmia	Deficiency of red blood cells

Using the Prefix, Root Word and Suffix To Form Words

Words can be formed by adding both the prefix and suffix to the root word.

Prefix	Root Word	Suffix	Combination	Definition
un-	sound	-ness	unSOUNDness	A horse's inability to walk or run correctly
PERi-	cardi-	-al	PERiCARdial	Area surrounding the heart
un-	DIlate	-ed	unDIlated	Not spread out, enlarged or expanded

Word Drill B

In the space provided, use the prefixes, suffixes, root words and combining forms from the list below to form the new word that corresponds to the definition given. The correct answers are listed in Appendix 1.

dys-: prefix meaning impaired or difficult.

POLy-: prefix meaning too much, in excess, many or multiple.

CRYo-: prefix pertaining to use of ultra-cold liquids.

MICro-: prefix meaning very small.

HYDro-: prefix pertaining to water.

-**EC**tomy: suffix meaning excision or removal of.

-**I**tis: suffix meaning inflammation of.

-**E**mia: suffix pertaining to blood.

-**U**ria: suffix pertaining to urine or urination.

-**PHA**gia: suffix pertaining to ingestion or swallowing.

-scope: suffix pertaining to an instrument for examination.

ARthr/o: combining form for joints.

HYSter/o: combining form pertaining to the uterus.

o**VAR**i/o: combining form pertaining to the ovary.

BLEPHar/o: combining form pertaining to the eyelids.

THERapy: word meaning treatment or nursing care.

SURgery: word meaning treatment by operative methods.

Example: Excision of the uterus: hyster/o plus -ectomy (drop the "o" because the suffix starts with a vowel) yields HYSter**EC**tomy.

1. Excision of the ovaries: _____

2. Excision of the uterus and ovaries: _____

3. Therapy involving water: _____

4. Surgery involving very small sites: _____

5. Inflammation of the heart: _____

6. Inflammation of the liver: _____

7. Production of excessive urine: _____

8. Surgery using ultracold temperatures to freeze tissues: ___

   _____

9. Instrument used to observe very small objects: _____

10. Difficulty in eating: _____

11. Spasms of the eyelids: _____

12. Knife used on a horse's hoof (compound word): _____

   _____

13. Disease of the foot causing the appearance of decay (compound word): _____

14. Inflammation of the bronchi: _____

15. Inflammation of multiple joints: _____

Defining Medical Terms by Word Analysis

So far, you have learned that by combining the component parts or elements in a systematic order, medical words with very specific meanings can be created. Words with precise meanings are vitally important in all areas of medicine, from describing findings on a pathology report to obtaining an accurate history for a patient.

If you understand how medical words are constructed, you can reverse the process in attempting to understand a medical word that is new to you. By breaking a word down into its component parts, you can determine the word's meaning.

How to systematically analyze medical words and determine their meaning is one of the skills you should achieve during your study of veterinary medical terminology. This ability also removes the mystery surrounding the long, seemingly complicated words so common to our profession. Word analysis makes medical terms easier to remember and encourages you to think logically.

How To Analyze Words

As mentioned above, the process of word analysis is the reverse of word construction. When analyzing a word, start at the end of the word (at the suffix) and work toward the prefix, analyzing the components in sequence.

Example: ovariohyster**EC**tomy = ovari o hyster ectomy.

                          4   3   2   1

1. The suffix "-ectomy" means to excise.

2. The root word "hyster-" refers to the uterus.

3. The "o" is the combining vowel for the previous root word.

4. The root word "ovari-" refers to the ovaries.

Thus, ovariohysterectomy means excision (removal) of the uterus and ovaries. Note that steps 3 and 4 could be combined into one step: The combining form "ovari/o" refers to the ovaries.

Some words, when analyzed, do not at first appear decipherable. Upon closer scrutiny, however, their meaning may become evident. Many of these words have an implied meaning rather than a literal one.

Example: di**SEASE** = dis (free of) + ease = free of ease.

Thus, an animal that is not at ease, then, must be ill or diseased.

Word analysis methodology does not work unfortunately with a number of words in veterinary medicine. Many of these words come from Latin, Greek or another language, and cannot be analyzed by the above method. The meaning of these words must simply be memorized.

When analyzing words, remember the various combining forms that pertain to the same anatomic part. This occurs because the combining forms are derived from both Latin and Greek.

Examples: cu**TA**ne/o, combining form for skin (Latin)

dermat/o, combining form for skin (Greek)

Also, even within the same language, various word elements may pertain to the same anatomic part.

Examples: hem/o, combining form for blood, as in he**MOL**ysis

hemat/o, combining form for blood, as in HEMa**TOL**ogy

Word Drill C

In the spaces provided, use word analysis to define the following medical words. The correct answers are listed in Appendix 1.

1. Polyunsaturated: _____

2. Hepatitis: _____

3. Hornfly:_____

4. Blepharitis:_____

5. Pericarditis: _____

6. Mastectomy: _____

7. Polyphagia:_____

8. Cryotherapy: _____

9. Arthroscope: _____

10. Hematuria: _____

Accents

The accented syllable is that part of a word that receives the most emphasis (by stress, pitch or both) during pronunciation. Listed below are rules for use of accents, as used in this text and in general.

Rules for Use of Accents

- In this book, accented syllables are printed in CAPITAL LETTERS. Syllables not accented are printed in small letters.

- In multisyllabic words with primary and secondary accents, the syllable with the primary (greater) accent is printed in **BOLDFACED CAPITAL LETTERS**, while the syllable with the secondary (lesser) accent is printed in CAPITAL LETTERS only. Unaccented syllables are printed in small letters. Multisyllabic words in which all syllables receive equal stress are printed in small letters.

    Example: inflammation: IN-fluh-**MAY**-shuhn

- In many cases, when adding a suffix in which the primary accent falls on a syllable of the suffix in the newly formed word, the secondary accent is then placed on the former primary accented syllable.

    Examples: e**SOPH**agus or e**SOPH**ag/o

eSOPHa**GO**tomy

- Medical words containing the suffixes listed below usually accent the third syllable from the end. The syllable accented in the following examples would be the combining vowel "o," which precedes the suffix. It is always a short "o" sound and is pronounced *ah*, as in pot.

-graphy	-lysis
-meter	-metry
-pathy	-phagy
-scopy	-logy

Example: bronchoscopy = brahn-**KAHS**-koh-pee

When the last 2 letters of a word or suffix are "-ia," the third syllable from the end is usually accented.

-Uria	**CAR**dia
-Emia	dys**TO**cia
-Algia	dys**LEX**ia
-PHAgia	aga**LAC**tia

The accent is placed on the second-to-last syllable: when the word contains only 2 syllables (atom); when the second-to-last syllable contains a diphthong (2 vowels written together and pronounced as a single vowel) (mouse pox); and when the suffix is one of the following:

-Ata	**-Osis**
-Atus	**-Oma**
-Atum	**-SO**ma
-Itis	**-Ura**

Pronunciation

Though many students find it difficult to pronounce medical words, it is important to learn how to correctly pronounce these terms. You may understand a word's meaning, but if you cannot pronounce it properly, you may be unable to effectively communicate with other medical personnel.

Pronunciation of medical terms may vary with the source consulted and a speaker's "natural" verbal accent. Phonetic spellings may differ among various dictionaries. The phonetic spellings used in this book are presented in a form readily understood by most students.

The following general rules will help you learn how to pronounce medical terms. As you proceed through the lessons, consult the glossary (Appendix 2) in the back of the book to learn pronunciations.

Vowel	Pronunciation
a	a (as in hat, can, bad)
	ah (as in hot, saw, ball)
	ahr (as in barn, far, star)
	air (as in bear, stair, hair)
	ay (as in day, hay, stay)
e	eh (as in let, step, yes)
	er (as in burn, manner, certain)
	ee (as in deed, see, be)
i	i (as in bit, tip, flip)
	eye (as in by, cry, fly)
	Note: When the long "i" is combined with other letters, it is written as "y," (as in byt, nyt, **SLYT**-lee). The long "i" is written as "eye" when it forms a syllable by itself (as in **EYE**-land).
o	oh (as in goat, go, boat)
	oo (as in do, group, boot)
	or (as in for, store, door)
	ow (as in cow, plow, now)
	oy (as in toy, joy, boy)
u	uh (as in pup, nut, run)
	uu (as in pull, full, good)
	yoo (as in you, cute, use)

Syllables

In this book, words have been divided into syllables to approximate the way they are pronounced, rather than according to standard rules of word division.

Accents

In the glossary (Appendix 2) and elsewhere throughout this book, accents are noted as follows:
- In multisyllabic words with primary and secondary accents, the syllable with the primary (greater) accent is printed in **BOLDFACED CAPITAL LETTERS**, while the syllable with the secondary (lesser) accent is printed in CAPITAL LETTERS only. Unaccented syllables are printed in small letters. For example, DER-muh-**TAH**-loh-jee.
- Syllables not accented are printed in small letters.
- Words of one syllable are printed in small letters. For example, host.
- Multisyllabic words in which all syllables receive equal stress are printed in small letters.

Pronouncing Vowels

Following are the phonetic spellings for pronunciation of vowels in medical terms.

Here are some general rules concerning vowels in medical terms.
- Generally, all vowels in scientific words are pronounced.
- Vowels can be short or long.
- An "a" at the end of a word usually is pronounced *uh,* as in idea.

Pronouncing Diphthongs

A diphthong consists of 2 adjacent vowels pronounced as a single vowel. Here are some general rules concerning pronunciation of diphthongs in medical terms.

- "ae" is pronounced *ee* (as in aeluropsis), except when followed by "r" or "s." "aer" is pronounced *air* (as in aerobic) and "aes" is pronounced *es* (as in aesthetic).
- "oe" is an English form in which the "o" is silent, so "oe" is pronounced *eh* (as in oestrus, written as estrus in North America).
- "oi" is pronounced *oy* (as in sarcoid).
- "eu" is pronounced *yoo* (as in eustachian).
- "ei" is pronounced *eye* (as in eisanthema).
- "ai" is pronounced *ay* (as in ailurophobia).
- "au" is pronounced *ah* (as in auditory).

Pronouncing Consonants

Following are pronunciations of consonants in medical terms.

Consonants	Pronunciation
b	as in boat, stable, crab
d	as in dark, fiddle, bed
f	as in fit, offer, stiff
h	as in house, ahead, behind
j	as in joy, magic, stage
k	as in can, action, back
l	as in leg, fully, pill
m	as in motor, stumble, trim
n	as in not, winner, fallen
ng	as in song, hanger, English
p	as in pill, wrapper, top
ph	as in photo, elephant, graph
r	as in rest, arrow, door
s	as in step, passive, brass
sh	as in sheer, mission, push
t	as in tip, better, boat
th	as in thin, thick, think
<u>th</u>	as in <u>th</u>em, <u>th</u>ere, <u>th</u>en
v	as in verse, oven, give
w	as in wall, wind, quick

x	as in tax, maximum, ax
z	as in zoo, crazy, freeze
zh	as in treasure, visual, measure

Here are some exceptions to the general rules concerning consonants in medical terms.

- "c" is pronounced as "k" at the end of a word (as in anemic) or if followed by "a," "o" or "u" (as in catheter).
- "c" is pronounced as "s" if followed by "e," "i" or "y" (as in cell).
- With "cc" followed by "i" or "y," the first "c" is pronounced as a "k" and the second as an "s" (as in accident).
- "ch" usually is pronounced as a "k" (as in chemistry).
- "cn" at the beginning of a word is pronounced as an "n" (as in cnidosis). Both letters are pronounced if "cn" appears in the middle of a word (as in gastrocnemius).
- "g" is pronounced as "j" if followed by "e," "i" or "y" (as in giant).
- "g" is pronounced as a hard "g" if followed by "a," "o" or "u" (as in gum).
- "gn" at the beginning or end of a word is pronounced as an "n" (as in gnat or benign). Both letters are pronounced if "gn" appears in the middle of a word (as in orthognathic).
- "mn" at the beginning of a word is pronounced as an "n" (as in mnemonic). Both letters are pronounced if "mn" appears in the middle of a word (as in amnesia).
- "pn" at the beginning of a word is pronounced as an "n" (as in pneumonia). Both letters are pronounced if "pn" appears in the middle of a word (as in dyspnea).
- "ps" at the beginning of a word is pronounced as an "s" (as in psychology). Both letters are pronounced if "ps" appears in the middle or end of a word (as in opsonin or cyclops).
- "pt" at the beginning of a word is pronounced as a "t" (as in ptosis). Both letters are pronounced if "pt" appears in the middle of a word (as in optical).
- "rh" is pronounced as "r" (as in rhinoceros).
- "th" may be pronounced as in "thin" or as in "then."

- "x" is pronounced as "z" at the beginning of a word (as in zero).

Word Drill D

In the space provided, spell each of the following words phonetically and label the primary (greater) accented syllable with 1 accent mark (') and the secondary (lesser) accented syllable with 2 accent marks ("). The correct answers are listed in the glossary (Appendix 2).

Example: hematology=hee"-muh-tah'-loh-jee

1. Gynecology: _____

2. Aerobic:_____

3. Euphoria: _____

4. Pneumonitis:_____

5. Phlebitis: _____

6. Chromosome:_____

7. Diarrhea: _____

8. Leiomyoma: _____

9. Aneurysm: _____

10. Cachexia:_____

11. Onychectomy: _____

12. Myoma: _____

13. Aplasia: _____

14. Ophthalmology:_____

15. Veterinary: _____

Tips on Studying Medical Terminology

- Try to thoroughly understand the methods of word construction and analysis, then study new medical words using these techniques.

- To understand any medical term, you must be able to define it, spell it correctly and pronounce it correctly. Correct pronunciation and spelling aid retention of the word and its meaning.
- When studying, correctly spell each word in writing, then pronounce and define it several times. Be particularly careful in spelling medical words. Changing a single letter can alter the entire meaning of a medical term. For example:
-
  ILium: one of the bones comprising the pelvis.

  ILeum: the distal portion of the small intestine.

- Make a set of flash cards (using 3 x 5-inch cards). On one side write the word and its phonetic spelling, and on the other side write the definition. For words that can be defined by word analysis, it may also be helpful to include that information on the card.
- Team up into pairs or form a study group to jointly make up flash cards and to quiz each other.
- Do not attempt to learn everything in each lesson in 1-2 days. Rather, study each lesson in increments. To retain this information, study and use the terms at every opportunity.
- Listen to the pronunciation of medical words by your instructor and others in the veterinary community.

Remember, how you are perceived by your peers, the doctors you work with and veterinary clients depends on how you express yourself. Understanding medical terminology is an important step toward becoming competent in your vocation.

Word Drill E

Using the clues provided on the following page, fill in the appropriate boxes. The correct answers are listed in Appendix 1.

Across

1. Inflammation of the mammary glands
2. Irritating dipterous insect
6. Suffix meaning degenerative condition
7. Suffix indicating inflammation
8. Abnormally low red blood cell count
10. Adjective for ox
13. Suffix related to blood
14. Practice of medicine on animals
18. An operation
19. Adjective for goats
20. Disease characterized by a rotting appearance of the feet
21. Adjective for horse
23. Nematodes that inhabit the blood vessel of horses
25. Prefix meaning water
26. Treatment
28. To breathe in
29. Suffix meaning the study of
30. Word termination that alters the meaning of words

Down

1. Adjective for mouse
2. Degenerative condition of the liver
3. Adjective for cat
4. Difficulty in urinating
5. Noun for avian
9. Illness or morbid process
11. To remove the horns
12. Slimy product of membranes
15. Study of words
16. Combining form for uterus
17. Instrument for examination
22. To breathe out
24. Noun for ovine
27. Prefix meaning many

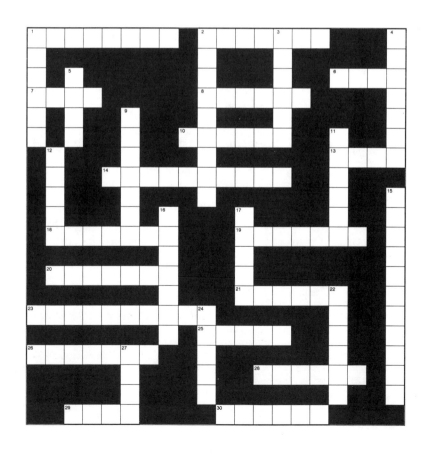

Lesson 2

Suffixes for Surgical Procedures

Lesson 1 showed that adding the suffix *-ectomy* to a combining form of a body part formed a word for a surgical procedure that meant excision or removal of that body part. The body part was indicated by the root word of the combining form.

Table 1 presents a list of suffixes for various surgical procedures. Using these suffixes as described above, you can form words to describe surgical procedures on various body parts, or define these words using the word analysis technique presented in Lesson 1.

Be careful with the spelling of the suffix *-rrhaphy*. It contains the letters "rrh," a common combination of letters in medical words. Other examples of words using "rrh" are hemorrhage and diarrhea.

Mispronunciation of medical words, especially ones with surgical suffixes, can lead to misspelling of these words. Regardless of how these surgical words might sound, their suffixes are always spelled the same. For example, tracheotomy may sometimes sound like tracheodomy, but the suffix is always spelled *"-tomy."*

Note: Throughout this book, syllables with a primary (greater) accent are printed in **BOLDFACED CAPITAL LETTERS**, while syllables with a secondary (lesser) accent are printed in CAPITAL LETTERS only. Unaccented syllables are printed in small letters.

Table 1. Suffixes for surgical procedures.

Suffix	Meaning	Example and Definition
-ECtomy	To excise or surgically remove	CHOlecys**TEC**tomy: surgical removal of the gallbladder
-tomy	To incise or cut into (make an incision)	lapaROTomy: surgical incision into the abdomen
-Stomy	To make a new opening in a hollow organ (to the outside of the body) or to make a new opening between 2 hollow organs	coLOStomy: surgical creation of a new opening from the colon to the outside of the body GAStroduode**NOS**tomy: to create a new opening from the stomach to the duodenum
-RRhaphy	To surgically repair by joining in a seam or by suturing together	HERni**ORR**haphy: surgical repair of a hernia
-PEXY	Fixation or suturing (a stabilizing type of repair)	**GAS**troPEXy: fixation of the stomach to the body wall
-PLASty	To shape or surgically form	**RHI**noPLASty: surgical reconstruction of the nose
-TRIPsy	To crush or destroy	**LITH**oTRIPsy: crushing of a stone (in the kidney, urinary bladder, or gallbladder); (lith/o= combining form meaning stone)
-cenTEsis	To puncture, perforate, permitting withdrawal of fluid or gas	abDOMinocen**TE**sis: surgical puncture of the abdomen to remove fluid from the peritoneal cavity

Later in this lesson you will have an opportunity to practice using these surgical suffixes by the techniques learned in Lesson 1 on word construction and word analysis. You will have to use the rules for combining forms when constructing new words using the surgical suffixes.

Root Words and Combining Forms for the Digestive System and Associated Structures

Table 2 presents a list of root words and their combining forms, corresponding to their associated body parts. Many of the body parts listed in Table 2 are defined in the glossary (Appendix 2). Because most of these words are derived from Latin or Greek, they will have to be memorized.

Note that some body parts have more than one combining form. Examples from Table 2 are:

mouth:	or/o, stomat/o
teeth:	dent/o, odont/o

This occurs because the combining forms originated from different languages, such as one from Latin and one from Greek. There are no general rules for when one or the other is used. This will have to be learned through listening and reading to be aware of how these combining forms are used. You already know some of them. For example, medication given by mouth is oral medication, not stomatal medication.

The different combining forms often refer to a specific part of a structure or specific use of a structure. For example, or/o often refers to the mouth as the start of the digestive system, whereas stomat/o refers to the lining of the oral cavity or the opening to the oral cavity (stomatitis, stomatoplasty).

A point of possible confusion is use of the words *abdominal* and *peritoneal*, and their respective cavities. The word *abdominal* is an adjective pertaining to the abdomen. The abdominal cavity contains the viscera (hollow organs) and the space between the organs and the body wall. The word *peritoneal* is an adjective pertaining to the peritoneum, which is the membranous lining on the inside of the body wall and covering the organs of the abdomen. The peritoneal cavity is the space between the organs and body wall. Therefore, the abdominal cavity is a combination of the peritoneal cavity and the organs of the abdomen.

Table 2. Combining forms for the digestive system.

Combining Form	Body Part
abDOMin/o	abdomen
aboMAS/o	abomasum
An/o	anus
CEc/o	cecum
CHEIl/o	lip
CHOl/o, chole-	bile
CHOleCYSt/o	gallbladder
CHOleDOch/o	common bile duct
cloAc/o	cloaca
COl/o	colon
COpr/o	feces
DENt/o	tooth, teeth
duOden/o	duodenum
ENter/o	intestines
eSOPHag/o	esophagus
GAStr/o	stomach
GINgiv/o	gingiva, gums
GLOSs/o	tongue
HEPa-, hePAT/o	liver
Ile/o	ileum
jeJUn/o	jejunum
LAPar/o	flank, abdomen
LINgua-, LINgu/o	tongue
oDONt/o	tooth, teeth
oMAs/o	omasum
Or/o	mouth
PALat/o	palate (hard or soft)
PANcreAt/o	pancreas
PERitoNE/o	peritoneum
PROCt/o	rectum
PROvenTRICul/o	proventriculus
pyLOr/o	pylorus
RECt/o	rectum
reTICul/o	reticulum
RUmen/o, RUmin/o	rumen
SIal/o	saliva, salivary glands
SPLANCHn/o	viscera
stoMAt/o	mouth
TONsill/o	tonsil
VIScer/o	viscera

If you are curious as to what types of surgeries are performed on the various body parts, consult your medical dictionary. Look in the section containing the root word of a body part in which you are interested. Observe the various suffixes attached. In addition to learning about the various surgeries performed, this will also teach you about the different diseases and conditions affecting that area of the body.

Word Drill A

Using word analysis, define each of the following words. Also write the phonetic spelling. The correct definitions are listed in Appendix 1. The phonetic spellings are listed in the glossary (Appendix 2).

1. gastrotomy: _____

_____

2. cholecystectomy: _____

_____

3. abomasopexy: _____

_____

4. rumenostomy: _____

_____

5. pyloroplasty: _____

_____

6. gastrojejunostomy: _____

_____

7. cholecystolithotripsy: _____

_____

8. enterotomy: _____

_____

9. hepatorrhaphy: _____

_____

10. rumenocentesis: _____

_____

Word Drill B

Using the definitions provided below, insert the correct medical word using the word construction techniques you have learned. The correct answers are listed in Appendix 1.

1. Surgical reconstruction of the mouth to improve function

   or appearance: _____

2. Incision into the esophagus: _____

3. Crushing of a stone in the intestine: _____

4. Removal of the tonsils: _____

5. Surgical fixation of the omasum: _____

6. Withdrawal of fluid from the common bile duct using a

   needle: _____

   _____

7. Surgical joining of the stomach to the intestines to create

   a new opening: _____

8. Surgical reconstruction of the lips to improve appearance:

   _____

9. Incision into the ileum: _____

10. Surgical removal of the pancreas: _____

Word Drill C: Important Words

The following words cannot be defined by word analysis. They must be memorized. Try to define each word, then look up the phonetic spelling and definition in the glossary (Appendix 2). Write the correct phonetic spellings and definitions in the spaces provided.

1. alimentary: _____

_____

2. alveolus: _____

_____

3. bloat:_____

_____

4. borborygmus: _____

_____

5. canine tooth: _____

_____

6. carnassial tooth: _____

_____

7. choke: _____

_____

8. coprophagy: _____

_____

9. defecation: _____

_____

10. emesis: _____

_____

11. entrails: _____

_____

12. eructate:_____

_____

13. eruption: _____

_____

14. excretion: _____

_____

15. feces: _____

_____

16. hernia: _____

_____

17. ileus: _____

_____

18. incisor: _____

_____

19. meconium: _____

_____

20. molar: _____

_____

21. peristalsis: _____

_____

22. premolar: _____

_____

23. scours: _____

_____

24. stool: _____

_____

25. viscus: _____

_____

Word Drill D

Using the clues provided on the following page, fill in the appropriate boxes. The correct answers are listed in Appendix 1.

Across

1. Cavity of the abdomen
2. Combining form for the pancreas
5. Combining form for the ileum
7. Combining form for the mouth
8. Root word for the tonsils
10. To belch gas
11. Common term for diarrhea
12. Suffix meaning to incise
15. Protrusion of tissues through an abnormal opening
17. Gaseous distention of the rumen
20. Suffix meaning to shape surgically
22. First stool of the newborn
24. Surgical repair of a hernia
27. Combining form for teeth
28. Visceral contractions
29. Combining form for feces
30. Singular form of the word viscera
31. A common term for feces

Down

1. The tract in which food passes from the mouth to the anus
2. The cavity between the viscera and the body wall
3. Suffix meaning to crush
4. Lack of contractile ability of a viscus
6. A tooth breaking through the gums
9. Medical word for the excrement from the bowels
13. Combining form for the saliva
14. To tap and withdraw fluid or gas
16. Surgical incision into the abdomen
18. Suffix meaning to make an artificial opening
19. Root word for bile
21. Suffix meaning a surgical fixation procedure
23. Colloquial term for foreign body in the esophagus
25. Vomiting
26. Body part for the combining form an/o

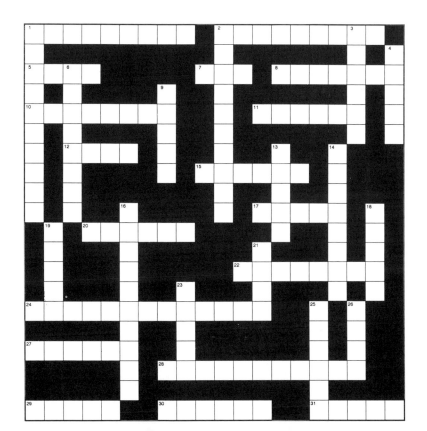

Lesson 3

Suffixes for Diseases
or Conditions

You have learned how to use the combining forms pertaining to organs and body parts together with surgical suffixes to form words describing surgical procedures on various body parts. The same procedure can be used with suffixes referring to diseases or conditions to describe a problem affecting a particular organ or body part. Table 1 presents a list of these suffixes.

As you can see from the list in Table 1, some of the definitions for the various suffixes are quite similar. The suffixes *-ia, -ism, -iasis, -itis, -osis* and *-pathy* refer to a disease or pathologic condition. Use of these word terminators, or suffixes, varies according to the type of disease, extent of damage, location, and if it is being used to name a disease or condition.

The suffix *-ia* is added to a root to form a word naming a specific disease or condition in which the location is indicated by the root word; for example, bacteriuria. A suffix describing a state or condition is *-ism;* for example, albinism. The suffix *-iasis* is used to form a word meaning a "condition characterized by." It is often used in parasitology to refer to infestation

Note: Throughout this book, syllables with a primary (greater) accent are printed in **BOLDFACED CAPITAL LETTERS,** while syllables with a secondary (lesser) accent are printed in CAPITAL LETTERS only. Unaccented syllables are printed in small letters.

Table 1. Suffixes for diseases or conditions.

Suffix	Meaning	Example and Definition
-ALgia or -DYnia	Pain	UreTHRALgia: pain in the urethra
-cele	Swelling, especially one with a cavity or hernia	RECtocele: hernial protrusion of a rectum (into the vagina).
-ECtasis or -ECtasia	Dilation, expansion or distention	GAStrecTAsia: dilation of the stomach.
-ia	A disease or condition, with location indicated by the root word.	BACteriURia: bacteria in the urine.
-Iasis	Infestation or infection of, or characterized by	ACaRIasis: infestation with mites.
-ISm	State, condition or result of a pathologic process	HYperCORticism: condition caused by an excess of glucocorticoids.
-Itis	Inflammation of	TONsilLItis: inflammation of the tonsils.
-Oma	Tumor	LEIomyOma: tumor of smooth muscles.
-Osis	Abnormal condition or process, often degenerative	nePHROsis: degenerative disease of the kidneys.
-pathy	Any disorder or disease condition	CARdiOPathy: disease of the heart.
-RRHAgia	Hemorrhage	RHInoRRHAgia: a bloody nose.

with external parasites or infection by internal parasites; for example, acariasis. The suffix *-osis* refers to a pathologic process and generally indicates a degenerative problem rather than an inflammatory one; for example, spondylosis. The word termination *-itis* is specific for an inflammatory problem; for example, phlebitis. The suffix *-pathy* is a more general term indicating disease in an organ, without specificity as to its nature; for example, cardiopathy.

The suffix -*sis* is of Greek origin and means a nonspecific state or condition. It generally appears with 1 or 2 vowels preceding it, such as in -*osis* and -*iasis*. These added vowels confer specific meanings. Other examples are -*esis* and -*asis;* -*esis* often refers to conditions involving the blood and sometimes urine, and -*asis* is not used frequently.

The suffix -*oma* usually refers to a benign growth or tumor, a type that does not spread to other parts of the body. In later lessons you will learn the words *carcinoma* and *sarcoma*, which are types of cancerous or malignant tumors.

Prefixes for Diseases or Conditions

Table 2 lists prefixes used to create words indicating the specific nature of a problem.

In Table 2, note that the prefix *py/o-* is written as a combining form. This means that it has a combining vowel "o," which may or may not be used. The example in Table 2, pyothorax, uses the combining vowel; however, the word pyuria (pus in the urine) does not. Another prefix in Table 2 also ends in "o" but is not written as a combining form. This is the prefix *hypo-*. When written as in Table 2, the letter "o" is always used in such prefixes. This format for listing prefixes is used in following lessons.

Root Words and Combining Forms for the Cardiovascular, Respiratory, Urinary and Reproductive Systems

Table 3 lists combining forms that correspond to their associated body parts.

As with Table 2 in Lesson 2, Table 3 also contains numerous combining forms for the same structure. Their uses often vary with the location to which the combining form refers. For example, *nephr/o* refers to the entire kidney, and conditions affecting the nephron. The combining form *ren/o* also refers to the entire kidney, while *pyel/o* refers to the pelvis of the kidney. Review the definitions in the glossary (Appendix 2) or

Table 2. Prefixes for diseases or conditions.

Prefix	Meaning	Example and Definition
a-, an-	Without or not having	aNEmia: not having enough red blood cells
ANti-	Against	ANtibiOTic: drug that acts against microorganisms
BRAdy-	Abnormally slow	BRAdyCARdia: abnormally slow heart rate
CONtra-	Against, opposed	CONtraINdicated: not to be performed or used
de-	Remove, take away, loss of	dehyDRAtion: excessive loss of body water
DIa-	Through, apart, across or between	DIaRRHEa: watery stool
dis-	Reversal or separation	diSEASE: illness
dys-	Difficult, impaired	dysPHAgia: difficulty eating or swallowing
HYper-	Excessive, abnormally high	HYperTHERmia: abnormally high body temperature
HYpo-	Insufficient, abnormally low	HYpoTHERmia: abnormally low body temperature
mal-	Bad, poor	maloCCLUsion: improper positioning of the teeth when the upper and lower arcades meet during chewing
PAth/o	Disease	paTHOLogy: the study of disease
POLy-	Many, much, multiple	POLyPHAgia: excessive eating
PY/o	Pus	PYoTHORax: pus in the thoracic or pleural cavity
TACHy-	Abnormally rapid	TACHyCARdia: abnormally rapid heart rate

Table 3. Combining forms pertaining to the cardiovascular, respiratory, urinary and reproductive systems.

Combining Forms	Examples	Body Parts
alVEol/o	alveolus	Teeth, lungs, mammary glands
ANgi/o	angiocarditis	Blood vessel
aORt/o	aortic	Aorta
arTERi/o	arterial	Artery
Atri/o	atrial	Atrium
BRONch/o, BRONchi-	bronchial	Bronchus
CARdi/o	cardiac	Heart
CERvic/o	cervix	Neck, uterus
CYSt/o	cystocentesis	Urinary bladder
CYt/o	cytologic	Cells
epiDIDym/o	epididymal	Epididymis
epiGLOTT/o	epiglottic	Epiglottis
ePISi/o	episioplasty	Vulva
HEm/o, heMAT/o	hemophilia	Blood
HYSTer/o	hysterectomy	Uterus
LAbi/o	labial	Lips, pudendum, labium
larYNg/o	laryngeal	Larynx
LOB/o	lobular	Lobe of lung, liver
MAST/o, MAMM/o	mammary	Mammary glands
MEtr/o	metrocele	Uterus
NEPHr/o	nephron	Kidney, nephron
ORchi/o, ORchid/o	orchiectomy	Testes
oVAri/o (OOPHor/o in people)	ovarian	Ovary
phaRYNG/o	pharyngeal	Pharynx
PHLEb/o	phlebolith	Veins
PLEUR/o	pleural	Pleura
PNEUm/o	pneumothorax	Lungs, air, breath
PROStat/o	prostatitis	Prostate gland
PULmo-, PULmon/o	pulmonary	Lungs
PYel/o	pyelitis	Pelvis of kidney
REn/o	renal	Kidney
RHIn/o	rhinoplasty	Nose
salPINg/o	salpingitis	Oviducts
SCROT/o	scrotal	Scrotum
SInus/o	sinusitis	Sinus
SPLEN/o	splenic	Spleen
STETH/o	stethomyositis	Chest
tesTICul/o	testicular	Testes
THORac/o	thoracic	Thorax
TRAche/o	tracheal	Trachea
uREter/o	ureteral	Ureters
uREthr/o	urethral	Urethra
Urin/o, Ur/o	urinary	Urine
Uter/o	uterine	Uterus
VAGin/o	vaginal	Vagina
VAS/o	vascular	Blood vessels
VEN/o	venous	Veins
venTRIcul/o	ventricular	Ventricle
VULv/o	vulvar	Vulva

your medical dictionary and observe the types of suffixes attached This will help you become more familiar with uses of these combining forms.

In Lesson 2 the words *abdominal* and *peritoneal* were explained. When referring to the chest, a similar relationship exists between the words *thoracic* and *pleural*, and their respective cavities. *Thoracic* is an adjective pertaining to the thorax. The thoracic cavity, like the abdominal cavity, contains organs and includes the space between the organs and the inner chest wall. *Pleural* is an adjective pertaining to the pleura, which is the membranous lining of the body wall and organs of the chest. The pleural cavity is the space between the organs, which is normally a vacuum and provides the negative pressure which allows the lungs to expand. The thoracic cavity is a combination of the pleural cavity and organs of the chest.

Another point of possible confusion is use of the terms *respiration* and *ventilation*. *Respiration* has 2 meanings: the act or function of breathing, sometimes called external respiration; and the transport of oxygen and carbon dioxide to and from the tissues, sometimes called internal respiration. *Ventilation* has several meanings: exchange of air between the lungs and the atmosphere (the mechanical process of respiration); the process of supplying oxygen to the lungs on a continual basis; and replacement of air in a room or building, generally by mechanical means. Respiration traditionally is used to indicate the physiologic process of breathing, whereas ventilation refers to the mechanical process of breathing.

Word Drill A

Using word analysis, define each of the following words and write the phonetic spelling in the space provided. The correct answers are listed in Appendix 1. Phonetic spellings are listed in Appendix 2. Compare the definitions you derived by word analysis to those in Appendix 2.

1. pyelonephritis:_____

2. aortectasia: _____

_____

3. bronchopneumonia: _____

_____

4. cystocele: _____

_____

5. cardiodynia: _____

_____

6. hepatoma: _____

_____

7. tracheopathy: _____

_____

8. urethrorrhagia: _____

_____

9. ureteropyosis: _____

_____

10. antidiarrheal: _____

_____

11. bradyphagia: _____

_____

12. polyuria: _____

_____

13. diapedesis (hint: "ped" means foot, walk, move): _____

_____

14. atelectasis (hint: "tela" means thin membrane): _____

_____

15. urolithiasis: _____

_____

Word Drill B

Using the definition provided below, supply the correct medical word in the space provided using the word construction techniques you have learned. You may have to use some word elements learned in Lessons 1 and 2. The correct answers are listed in Appendix 1.

1. Inflammation of the prostate gland: _____

2. Dilation of the bronchi: _____

3. Inflammation of the vulva and vagina:_____

4. Abnormal presentation of the fetus in the birth canal:____

_____

5. Inflammation of multiple sinuses: _____

6. Degenerative condition of the kidney's nephrons: _____

_____

7. Pain in the bladder: _____

8. Bleeding from the uterus: _____

9. Difficulty in urination:_____

10. Disease of the kidneys:_____

11. Infection with ascarids (ascar-): _____

12. Abnormally rapid respiration (hint: use -pnea as suffix):__

_____

13. Inflammation of the uterus, with the presence of pus: ____

_____

14. Excessive sensitivity to pain: _____

15. Low motility (of the gut): _____

Word Drill C

This drill requires use of the information you have learned in the previous lessons. With the definitions provided, write the correct medical word using the word construction techniques you have learned. The correct answers are listed in Appendix 1.

1. Inflammation of the stomach: _____

2. Incision into the trachea: _____

3. Crushing a stone in the pelvis of the kidney: _____

_____

4. Surgical removal of the spleen: _____

5. Degenerative condition of the liver: _____

6. Bloat or dilation of the rumen: _____

7. Inflammation of the colon: _____

8. Surgical fixation of the uterus: _____

9. Surgical removal of the testes: _____

10. Toothache: _____

Word Drill D

The following words, related to diseases of the cardiovascular, respiratory, urinary and reproductive systems, cannot be defined by word analysis. Try to define each word, then look up the phonetic spelling and definition in the glossary (Appendix 2). Write the correct phonetic spellings and definitions in the spaces provided.

1. abort: _____

_____

2. acute: _____

_____

3. afterbirth: _____

_____

4. aneurysm: _____

_____

5. barren: _____

_____

6. breech: _____

_____

7. calculus: _____

_____

8. chronic: _____

_____

9. copulation: _____

_____

10. ecchymosis: _____

_____

11. epistaxis: _____

_____

12. exacerbation: _____

_____

13. gestation: _____

_____

14. grave: _____

_____

15. gravid: _____

_____

16. heat: _____

_____

17. inbreeding: _____

_____

18. incontinent: _____

_____

19. inflammation: _____

_____

20. intact: _____

_____

21. micturition: _____

_____

22. parturition: _____

_____

23. petechia:_____

_____

24. pseudocyesis:_____

_____

25. urination:_____

_____

Word Drill E

Using the clues provided on the following page, fill in the appropriate boxes. The correct answers are listed in Appendix 1.

Across

1. Condition characterized by stone formation
3. Relating to the chest cavity
6. Suffix meaning excessive flow
8. Prefix meaning without
9. Definition of the prefix py/o
10. Common name for estrus
13. Medical word for stone
14. Not surgically neutered
15. Prefix meaning opposite
16. Suffix referring to an infestation or infection
17. Suffix for any disorder of an organ or system
20. Persisting over a long period
21. Prefix meaning against
22. Prefix meaning insufficient
26. Prefix meaning difficult or impaired
28. Medical word for giving birth
31. Malpresentation in which the fetal rear end emerges first
32. Body part for the combining form cardi/o

33. Tissue reaction causing redness, heat, swelling and pain
34. To expel a fetus before term
35. Abnormally rapid heart rate
36. Suffix meaning a degenerative condition

Down

1. Combining form for the larynx
2. Mechanical process of breathing
4. Suffix meaning tumor
5. Sexual union
7. Suffix meaning pain
11. Period from conception to birth
12. Prefix meaning bad, poor or abnormal
14. Suffix meaning inflammation of
18. Abnormally high body temperature
19. Physiologic process of breathing
23. Pus in the thoracic cavity
24. Prefix meaning abnormally slow
25. Meaning of the combining form pneum/o
27. Inflammation of the sinuses
29. Combining form referring to the kidney
30. Combining form referring to the uterus

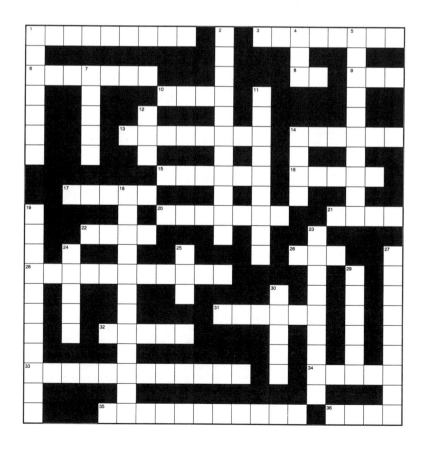

Lesson 4

Plural Endings

It is important to understand the methods for converting singular forms of medical words to their plural forms. Table 1 lists common singular endings and their corresponding plural endings.

Not every word ending in -*us* has a plural form that ends in -*i*. For example, the plural form of "sinus" is "sinuses," not "sini." There is no rule for which plurals end in -*i* and which ones end in -*es*. These distinctions must be learned with use or by consulting your medical dictionary.

Table 1. Singular and plural word endings.

Singular	Plural	Examples
-a	-ae	VERtebra, VERtebrae
-anx	-anges	PHAlanx, phaLANges
-en	-ina	LUmen, LUmina
-ex, -ix	-ices	Apex, Apices
		CERvix, CERvices
-is	-es	TEStis, TEStes
-inx	-inges	MENinx, meNINges
-ma	-mata or -mas	ENema, eneMAta or ENemas
-um	-a	Ovum, Ova
-ur	-ora	FEmur, FEMora
-us	-i	Uterus, Uteri

Note: Throughout this book, syllables with a primary (greater) accent are printed in **BOLDFACED CAPITAL LETTERS**, while syllables with a secondary (lesser) accent are printed in CAPITAL LETTERS only. Unaccented syllables are printed in small letters.

Word Drill A

Write the plural form and phonetic spelling for each of the following words in the space provided. The correct answers are listed in the glossary (Appendix 2). If you do not know the meaning of a word, read its definition in Appendix 2 when checking your answers.

1. bursa:_____

_____

2. serum: _____

_____

3. nucleus:_____

_____

4. diagnosis: _____

_____

5. appendix:_____

_____

6. carcinoma: _____

_____

7. meniscus: _____

_____

8. foramen: _____

_____

9. speculum: _____

_____

Word Drill B

Write the singular form and phonetic spelling for each of the following words in the space provided. The correct answers are listed in the glossary (Appendix 2). If you do not know the meaning of a word, read the definition in Appendix 2 when you are checking your answers.

1. atria: _____

_____

2. data: _____

_____

3. foci: _____

_____

4. prognoses: _____

_____

5. sarcomata: _____

_____

6. laminae: _____

_____

7. gingivae:_____

_____

8. fornices: _____

_____

9. gyri:_____

_____

10. syringes: _____

_____

Root Words and Combining Forms for the Musculoskeletal, Integumentary, Nervous, Endocrine and Lymphatic Systems and Associated Structures

This is the final lesson in which you will learn root words and their combining forms for associated body parts. Table 2 lists their combining forms for the musculoskeletal, integumentary, nervous, endocrine and lymphatic systems.

Table 2. Combining forms pertaining to the musculoskeletal, integumentary, nervous, endocrine and lymphatic systems.

Combining Form	Body Part
AceTABul/o	acetabulum
ADen/o	gland
ADip/o	fat
adREn/o, adREnal-	adrenal gland
ARthr/o	joint
axILL/o	axilla
BLEPHar/o	eyelid, eyelash
burs/o	bursa
CANth/o	canthus
CARp/o	carpus
CEPHal/o	head
cereBELL/o	cerebellum
ceREbr/o	cerebrum
CHONdr/o	cartilage
CHORD/o	spinal cord
COCCYg/o	coccyx
CONjuncTIv/o	conjunctiva
COST/o	rib
COX/o	hip, pelvis
CRAni/o	cranium, skull
DERm/o, derMAt/o	skin
desceMET/o	descemet's membrane
enCEPHal/o	brain
ePIPHys/o, epiPHYSi/o	epiphysis
FEmor/o	femur
FIBul/o	fibula
GNATH/o	jaw
HISt/o	tissue
HUmer/o	humerus
ILi/o	ilium
Ir-, IRid/o	iris
ISchi/o	ischium
KERat/o	cornea, horny tissue
LAMin/o	lamina, flat part of a vertebra
LIP/o	fat
lymPHADen/o	lymph node
LYMphang/o, lymPHANgi/o	lymph vessel
LYMPH/o	lymph
manDIBul/o	mandible
MAXill/o	maxilla
meNINg/o	meninges
meNISC/o	meniscus
MUScul/o, MY/o, MYos-	muscle
MYel/o	bone marrow or spinal cord
myRING/o	ear drum
NEUR/o	nerve

(Table 2 continued)

Combining Form	Body Part
OCul/o	eye
ONych/o	claw, hoof
ophTHALm/o	eye
OSte/o	bone
Ot/o	ear
paraTHYr/o	parathyroid gland
PELvi/o, PELv/o	pelvis
PIl/o	hair
POd/o, PEd/o	foot
PUB/o	pubis
RAdi/o	radius
RETin/o	retina
SAcr/o	sacrum
SCAPul/o	scapula
SCLER/o	sclera, or hard
SPONdyl/o	vertebra, spinal column
STERn/o	sternum
synDESm/o	ligament, connective tissue
syNOvi/o	synovium, synovial fluid
TARs/o	tarsus
TEN/o, TENd/o, TENdin/o	tendon
THYr/o	thyroid gland
TIBi/o	tibia
TYMpan/o	tympanum (middle ear), tympanic
ULn/o	ulna
Uve/o	uvea
VERtebr/o	vertebra

The combining forms for skeletal parts are not often used to make medical words that describe a disease or specific surgery. For example, veterinarians do not usually do an ulnectomy. Inflammation of the fibula is not described as fibulitis, but rather as osteitis of the fibula. The purpose of this is to specifically describe the nature of the bone disease. However, combining forms are often used when describing joints. For example, the hip joint is called the coxofemoral joint.

Word Drill C

Using word analysis, define each of the following medical words and write their phonetic spellings in the space provided.

The correct answers are listed in Appendix 1. The phonetic spellings are listed in the glossary (Appendix 2). Remember to compare your definitions to those in the glossary.

1. spondylosis: _____

_____

2. parathyroidectomy:_____

_____

3. lipoma:_____

_____

4. neurotripsy: _____

_____

5. laminectomy: _____

_____

6. myringoplasty:_____

_____

7. encephalitis: _____

_____

8. dermatosis: _____

_____

9. craniotomy:_____

_____

10. descemetocele: _____

_____

Word Drill D

From the definitions below, use the word construction techniques you have learned and write the correct medical word in the space provided. Correct answers are listed in Appendix 1.

1. Incision into the pyloric musculature: _____

2. Removal of the claws of a cat:_____

3. Disease of the nerves: _____

4. Inflammation of the meninges: _____

5. Inflammation of a tendon's synovial membranes: _____

_____

6. Joint formed by the tibia and the tarsus: _____

_____

7. Inflammation of more than one joint: _____

8. Surgical removal of a meniscus: _____

9. Disease of the lymph nodes: _____

10. Inflammation of the bone and bone marrow: _____

_____

11. Inflammation of the muscles: _____

12. Study of pathology of tissues: _____

13. Inflammation of the cornea: _____

14. Junction between the bony rib and the cartilage portion
    of the rib: _____

15. Surgical removal of fat: _____

Word Drill E: Important Words

The following words, related to the muscles, nerves, skin, glands, lymphatics, eye or ear, generally cannot be defined by word analysis. Try to define each word, then look up the phonetic spelling and definition in the glossary (Appendix 2). Write the correct phonetic spelling and definitions in the spaces provided.

1. appendage: _____

_____

2. articular: _____

_____

3. cannon bone: _____

_____

4. cataract: _____

_____

5. chestnut: _____

_____

6. coffin bone or joint: _____

_____

7. conformation: _____

_____

8. dewclaw: _____

_____

9. digit: _____

_____

10. ergot: _____

_____

11. false ribs: _____

_____

12. fetlock joint: _____

_____

13. hock: _____

_____

14. miosis: _____

_____

15. mydriasis: _____

_____

16. navicular: _____

_____

17. palpebra: _____

_____

18. pastern bones and joints: _____

_____

19. pinna: _____

_____

20. process: _____

_____

21. quick: _____

_____

22. sesamoid bones: _____

_____

23. sprain: _____

_____

24. stifle joint: _____

_____

25. tubercle: _____

_____

Word Drill F

Using the clues provided on the following page, fill in the appropriate boxes. The correct answers are listed in Appendix 1.

Across

1. Plural form for meninx
3. Dilation of the pupils
4. Combining form for nerves
5. Combining form for cartilage
10. The knee joint
12. Combining form for bone
14. Combining form for the eye
15. Singular of gyri
16. Sensitive part of the nail or claw
20. Iris, ciliary body and choroid layer
22. Body part of the combining form irid/o
23. Plural of foramen
25. Collapse of sections of lung
28. Singular of femora
29. Combining form for lymph vessels
30. Inflammation of the kidney
31. Eyelid

Down

1. Excision of a meniscus
2. The ear flap
3. Combining form for eardrum
6. Benign fatty tumor
7. Plural of vertebra
8. Combining form for tissue
9. Opacity of the lens
11. Constriction of the pupils
13. The hip joint
17. Excision of a lamina
18. Singular of ova
19. Singular of bursae
21. Body part for the combining form gnath/o
24. Body part for the combining form kerat/o
26. Body part for the combining form ot/o
27. Horny material distal to the fetlock
29. Body part for the combining form labi/o

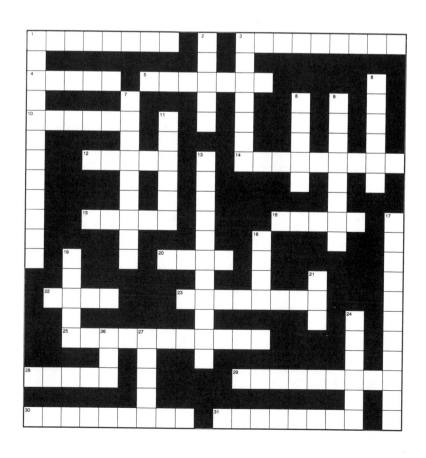

Lesson 5

Instruments and Procedures

Table 1 lists suffixes that, when added to a combining form of a body part, form a word pertaining to an instrument or piece of equipment used to examine, section or measure that body part.

An instrument used for viewing is a SPECulum. This instrument is used to hold open a passage or cavity so that the veterinarian can observe the interior. The long and narrow attachments for an otoscope, which are placed inside the ear canal to facilitate viewing, are the specula (plural of speculum) for the otoscope.

Generally, instruments that end with "-scope" have a light source that allows the veterinarian to view inside the canal or opening as the scope is inserted. For example, otoscope. Not all scopes are used for viewing. For example, the scope below is used for listening.

STETHoscope: instrument used for auscultation of the thorax and abdomen.

One method of remembering that the suffix *"-tome"* refers to cutting is by recalling that the suffix *"-tomy"* means to in-

Note: Throughout this book, syllables with a primary (greater) accent are printed in **BOLDFACED CAPITAL LETTERS**, while syllables with a secondary (lesser) accent are printed in CAPITAL LETTERS only. Unaccented syllables are printed in small letters.

cise or cut into. They both originate from the same Greek word *tome*, which means to cut.

When pronouncing -(O)Scopy and -(O)Graphy, the primary accented syllable is the third from the last, whereas in words ending in *-scope* or *-graph,* the primary accented syllable is farther forward in the words.

Table 1. Suffixes related to instruments and equipment.

Suffix	Meaning	Example and Definition
-scope	Instrument for examining. such as viewing or listening	Otoscope: instrument for looking into the ears
-scopy	The act of examining or using the scope	LAPaROScopy: procedure of using a laparoscope to view the abdominal cavity
-tome	Instrument for cutting	OSteotome: instrument for cutting bone
-graph	Instrument or machine that writes or records	eLECtroCARdiograph: machine that records the electrical impulses generated by the heart
-graphy	Procedure of using an instrument or machine to record	eLECtroCARdiOGraphy: procedure of using an electrocardiograph to produce an electrocardiogram
-gram	The product, written record, "picture" or graph produced by an instrument	eLECtroCARdiogram: linear tracing of the electrical impulses generated by the heart
-meter	Instrument or machine that measures or counts	therMOMeter: instrument used to measure temperature
-metry -IMetry	Procedure of measuring	doSIMetry: act of determining the amount, rate and distribution of ionizing radiation

There is not always a special machine for various procedures. For example, myelography, in which radiopaque dye is injected into the subarachnoid space and radiographs made, is performed using an ordinary x-ray machine.

An exception to the rules listed above involves use of the word "radiograph." According to Table 1, a radiograph would be an instrument or machine; however, we know the instrument is an x-ray machine. The word radiograph means the same as radiogram, the image produced on radiographic film. In fact, radiograph is the more commonly used word.

Word Drill A

Using word analysis, define each of the following medical words and write their phonetic spelling in the spaces provided. The correct answers are listed in Appendix 1. The phonetic spellings are listed in the glossary (Appendix 2). Remember to compare your definitions to those in the glossary.

1. electroencephalography: _____

_____

2. echocardiogram: _____

_____

3. dermatome: _____

_____

4. ophthalmoscope: _____

_____

5. cystoscopy: _____

_____

6. pelvimetry: _____

_____

7. arthroscope: _____

_____

8. tonometer (hint: tono- is from the root *tone*, or pressure): _

_____

_____

9. spirometry (hint: spiro-, from the Latin word *spirare,*

means to breathe): _____

_____

10. gastroscope: _____

_____

Word Drill B

In the spaces provided, write the medical word for the instrument, act, procedure or record indicated by each definition. The correct answers are listed in Appendix 1.

1. Instrument for recording muscle contractions:_____

_____

2. Procedure of looking into a joint:_____

3. Radiographic image produced on film after radiopaque

dye is injected into the spinal canal: _____

4. Radiographic image produced on film after radiopaque

dye is injected into a blood vessel: _____

5. Instrument used to make micro-thin tissue slices:_____

_____

6. Radiographic image produced on film by radiography

of the mammary glands:_____

7. Instrument that counts cell numbers

(hint: cyt/o refers to cell):_____

8. Instrument for dilating the vagina for examination

(hint: answer is 2 words):_____

9. Procedure of viewing the colon: _____

10. Instrument used to view the bronchi: _____

Word Drill C

The following words have some relationship to surgical and medical instruments. These words generally cannot be defined by word analysis. Try to define each word, then look up the phonetic spelling and definition in the glossary (Appendix 2). Write the correct phonetic spellings and definitions in the spaces provided.

1. aperture: _____

_____

2. arrhythmia: _____

_____

3. aspirate: _____

_____

4. autoclave: _____

_____

5. balling gun: _____

_____

6. barrier: _____

_____

7. biopsy: _____

_____

8. catheter: _____

_____

9. cautery: _____

_____

10. declaw: _____

_____

11. elastrator: _____

_____

12. Elizabethan collar: _____

_____

13. emasculatome: _____

_____

14. emasculator: _____

_____

15. graft: _____

_____

16. hemostat: _____

_____

17. restraint: _____

_____

18. scalpel: _____

_____

19. sphygmomanometer: _____

_____

20. splint: _____

_____

21. stitch: _____

_____

22. suture: _____

_____

23. swage: _____

_____

24. twitch: _____

_____

25. Wood's light: _____

_____

Word Drill D

Using the clues provided on the following page, fill in the appropriate boxes. The correct answers are listed in Appendix 1.

Across

1. Instrument for looking into the ear
2. Instrument for measuring pressure inside the eye
6. Instrument for recording electrical impulses generated by the heart
9. Instrument for listening to the chest
12. Material used to close wounds
13. Suffix for an instrument used for examining
14. Transfer of tissue from one site to another
17. Radiograph of dye injected into the subarachnoid space surrounding the spinal cord
21. Suffix for an instrument that measures
23. Surgical removal of a piece of tissue for analysis
24. Instrument used to clamp bleeding blood vessels
25. Tube placed into a vessel, viscus or cavity to withdraw or administer fluids
26. Prodcedure for viewing the interior of the abdomen

Down

1. Instrument used to cut bone
2. Instrument used to measure temperature
3. Instrument used to measure blood pressure
4. Suffix for a cutting instrument
5. Instrument used to dilate an orifice to allow viewing
7. Instrument used to castrate large animals by crushing the spermatic cord
8. Combining form for ear
10. Suffix referring to a tumor, swelling or cavity
11. Act of measuring the pelvic canal
15. Restraint device placed on the upper lip of horses
16. Suffix referring to an instrument that records
18. Common name for sutures in a wound
19. Suffix for the recording produced by an instrument
20. Suffix meaning the act of examining (with an instrument)
22. Application of an agent or instrument to stop bleeding

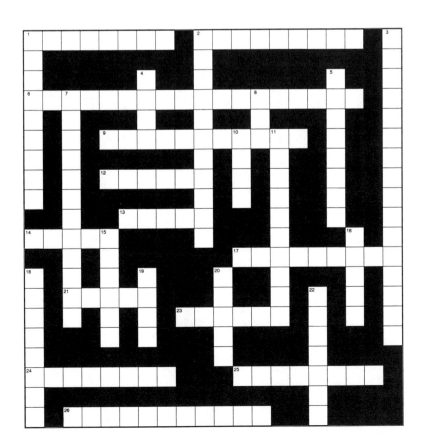

Lesson 6

Suffixes and Titles for the Medical Disciplines

The suffix *"-logy"* (from the Greek *logos,* meaning reason) is a word termination meaning "the science of" or "the study of." The subject is designated by the root word to which the suffix is attached. So far in this text you have been introduced to the following:

Subject	Definition
TERmiNOLogy	study of words
paTHOLogy	study of the nature of disease
CARdiOLogy	study of the heart and its diseases
psyCHOLogy	study of the mind
HEMaTOLogy	study of blood and its diseases

A person who studies or practices a specific science is referred to by attaching the suffix *"-logist"* to the root word on which the science is based. Examples based on these subjects are listed below.

Subject	Practitioner
terminology	TERmiNOLogist

> Note: Throughout this book, syllables with a primary (greater) accent are printed in **BOLDFACED CAPITAL LETTERS**, while syllables with a secondary (lesser) accent are printed in CAPITAL LETTERS only. Unaccented syllables are printed in small letters.

Subject	Practitioner
pathology	paTHOLogist
cardiology	CARdiOLogist
psychology	psyCHOLogist
hematology	HEMaTOLogist

When the word *medicine* is used, it refers to all forms of medicine, such as veterinary, human, dental and osteopathic.

Other suffixes refer to persons that study or practice a particular science. These suffixes mean the same as *"-logist"* (Table 1).

Note from the definitions in Table 1 that for a branch of medicine ending in the suffix *"-try,"* the suffix *"-iatrist"* is used to denote a practitioner. Similarly, for a branch of medicine that ends in *"-ic,"* the suffix *"-ician"* is used to denote a practitioner. Other examples are:

Subject	Practitioner
obstetrics	OBsteTRIcian
podiatry	poDIatrist

Another term related to the practice of medicine is the word *iatrogenic*, which describes a condition in a patient resulting from treatment by a veterinarian (or a practitioner in another field of medicine). The suffix *"-iatrist"* and the prefix *"iatro-"* evolved from the same Greek word *iatros*, meaning physician.

Table 1. Alternative terms used for practitioners of various sciences.

Suffix	Example	Definition
-ist	inTERnist	One who practices internal medicine
-Iatrist	psyCHIatrist	One who practices psychiatry, treating disorders of the psyche
-ICian	PEdiaTRICian	One who practices pediatrics
-er -(Itioner)	pracTItioner	One who practices in a profession, especially medical sciences

Thus, the word *iatrogenic*, as defined by word analysis, means originating from a physician (*iatro* = physician and *-genic* = origin of, from the word *genesis*).

There are many different types of a doctorate degree. Not all recipients are "DOCtors" in the classic use of the term, in which it is synonymous with the word physician. To be addressed as "doctor," a doctorate degree is required. Table 2 lists some examples of doctorate degrees.

Specialty Areas and Specialists

Veterinary medicine, like human medicine, has areas of specialization. Specialists usually spend 3-5 years of study in their specialty field at a university teaching hospital before taking their specialty board examinations. Upon passing these examinations, they become "members" or "diplomates" of the

Table 2. Types of doctorate degrees.

Degree	Definition
DVM or VMD	**Doctor of Veterinary Medicine**: a veterinarian.
MD	**Doctor of Medicine**: a physician.
DO	**Doctor of Osteopathy**: an osteopathic physician.
DMD or DDS	**Doctor of Dental Medicine or Doctor of Dental Surgery**: a dentist.
DC	**Doctor of Chiropractic Medicine**: a chiropractor; treats with manipulative therapy, may use radiography.
OD	**Doctor of Optometry**: an optometrist; treats refractive errors, fits eyeglasses; differs from an ophthalmologist, which is a veterinarian, physician or osteopath who specializes in the diagnosis and treatment of disorders of the eye.
DPM	**Doctor of Podiatry**: a podiatrist; specializes in care of the feet, including radiography, surgery, various therapies and medication.
PhD	**Doctor of Philosophy**: can be granted in any field of study, from history to religion, to a postdoctoral specialty degree in ophthalmology. These people are also addressed as "doctor" but sometimes are called "professor," as most of the professors at colleges and universities have this degree.

College or Board of their particular specialty. Veterinarians who become specialists generally obtain a postdoctoral master's degree or PhD in their specialty (this differs from human medicine).

Following is a list of veterinary specialty areas and specialists, and a brief description of what they do. In some of these areas there is no specialty board yet, or they are classified as specialists within the specialty board of internal medicine.

ANesTHEsiOLogy, ANesTHEsiOLogist: the study of administration of drugs to induce narcosis and/or analgesia for performing surgery and other procedures, so as to eliminate pain. The "aNESthetist" differs from the anesthesiologist, who is a DVM or MD. The anesthetist is a licensed veterinary technician, or registered nurse who has attended a nurse anesthetist school.

CARdiOLogy, CARdiOLogist: the study of the heart and blood vessels (cardiovascular disorders and cardiovascular surgery). In veterinary medicine it is a subspecialty of internal medicine.

DERmaTOLogy, DERmaTOLogist: the study of disorders of the skin.

ENdocriNOLogy, ENdocriNOLogist: the study of disorders of ductless or endocrine glands, which produce hormones (for example, the thyroid gland). In veterinary medicine, it is a division of internal medicine.

GAStroENterOLogy, GAStroENterOLogist: the study of disorders of the stomach and intestines. In veterinary medicine it is a division of internal medicine.

InTERnal MEDicine, InTERnist: the study of disorders of internal body systems, divided into subspecialties of cardiology, internal medicine, neurology, and oncology. In veterinary medicine it is also sometimes divided between large and small animals.

LABoraTOry ANimal MEDicine, **LAB**oraTOry ANimal SPEcialist: the study of disorders of laboratory animals, such as rats, mice, rabbits, gerbils, hamsters, guinea pigs, dogs, cats, ferrets and subhuman primates.

MIcrobiOLogy, MIcrobiOLogist: the study of microorganisms, such as bacteria, viruses and fungi.

NeuROLogy, neuROLogist: the study of disorders of the brain, spinal cord and nerves. In veterinary medicine it is a subspecialty of internal medicine.

ObSTETrics and GYneCOLogy, OBsteTRICian, GYneCOLogist: the study of disorders of the female reproductive tract, prenatal care, parturition (birth), postpartum care, gynecologic surgery and some urinary tract infections. A specialty only in human medicine.

OnCOLogy, onCOLogist: the study of tumors and cancer, including radiation therapy, surgery and chemotherapy of tumors. It is a specialty of veterinary internal medicine.

OPHthalMOLogy, OPHthalMOLogist: the study of disorders of the eye.

OtoRHInoLARynGOLogy, OtoRHInoLARynGOLogist: the study of disorders of the ear, nose and throat.

PaTHOLogy, paTHOLogist: the study of the causes and effects of disease on the structure and function of tissues and organs; includes microscopic and macroscopic (gross or with the unaided eye) examination of tissues; also divided into clinical pathology, which includes hematologic (blood disorders) and blood chemistry analysis.

PEdiATrics, PEdiaTRICian: the study of disorders of young animals or children under 16 years old.

PsyCHIatry, psyCHIatrist: the study of disorders of the mind; a post-MD specialty with no veterinary equivalent.

PsyCHOLogy, psyCHOLogist: the study of the mind and mental processes, especially in regard to behavior; psychologists are not allowed to dispense or prescribe medicine and generally have a master's degree and/or PhD in the field of psychology; though this is not a specialty area of veterinary medicine, some veterinarians have studied animal psychology and are well versed in the subject.

RAdiOLogy, RAdiOLogist: the study of use of irradiation in the diagnosis and treatment of disease.

SURgery, SURgeon: the study of treatment of disease by operative methods; general surgery is divided into such areas as neurosurgery, orthopedic surgery (bones and joints), plastic surgery, thoracic surgery and vascular surgery; in veterinary medicine it is also divided according to large and small animal emphasis.

THERiogenOLogy, THERiogenOLogist: the study of reproduction and reproductive disorders of animals.

TOXiCOLogy, TOXiCOLogist: the study of poisons and the disorders they cause.

UROLogy, uROLogist: the study of disorders of the urinary tract; in veterinary medicine it is a division of internal medicine; in human medicine it also includes the male reproductive tract.

ZOoLOGic MEDicine, ZOoLOGic MEDicine SPEcialist: the study of disorders of zoo animals, and wild and exotic species.

Word Drill A

Define the following terms. The correct answers are listed in the glossary (Appendix 2).

1. specialist: _____

_____

2. practitioner: _____

_____

3. intern: _____

_____

4. internist: _____

_____

5. resident: _____

Word Drill B

Name the specialist that would treat a patient with the following conditions. The correct answers are listed in Appendix 1. Look up the phonetic spellings in the glossary (Appendix 2) to be sure you can pronounce these words correctly.

1. urinary tract infection: _____

2. ear infection: _____

3. fractured leg: _____

4. heart problems: _____

5. epilepsy: _____

6. cataracts: _____

7. skin infection: _____

8. dystocia: veterinary medicine: _____

          human medicine: _____

9. stomach ulcers: _____

10. cause of poisoning: _____

Word Drill C

Name the specialty area that deals with the following organs, species, or organisms. The correct answers are listed in Appendix 1. Look up the phonetic spellings in the glossary (Appendix 2) to be sure you can pronounce these words correctly.

1. parathyroid gland: _____

2. red blood cells: _____

3. monkeys: _____

4. turkeys: _____

5. tumors: _____

6. dead animals: _____

7. spinal cord problems: _____

8. fracture repair: _____

9. *Staphylococcus* bacteria: _____

10. corneal ulcers: _____

Word Drill D: Important Words

The following medical terms are associated with diagnostic and surgical procedures performed by veterinarians and, in some cases, technicians under supervision of a veterinarian. These words generally cannot be defined by word analysis. Try to define each word, then look up the phonetic spelling and definition in the glossary (Appendix 2). Write the correct phonetic spellings and definitions in the spaces provided.

1. anastomosis: _____

_____

2. asymptomatic: _____

_____

3. auscultation: _____

_____

4. castrate: _____

_____

5. cut: _____

_____

6. debride: _____

_____

7. dock: _____

_____

8. enema: _____

_____

9. enucleation: _____

_____

10. eviscerate: _____

_____

11. float: _____

_____

12. gavage: _____

_____

13. geld: _____

_____

14. intubate: _____

_____

15. lance: _____

_____

16. necropsy: _____

_____

17. neuter: _____

_____

18. palpation: _____

_____

19. paracentesis: _____

_____

20. percussion: _____

_____

21. resection: _____

_____

22. signs: _____

_____

23. spay: _____

_____

24. symptoms: _____

_____

25. tap: _____

_____

Word Drill E

Using the clues provided on the following page, fill in the appropriate boxes. The correct answers are listed in Appendix 1.

Across

1. Act of controlling or restricting movement
2. Practitioner of internal medicine
4. To remove dead or necrotic material from a wound
6. Slang term for the act of castration
7. Common term for withdrawal of fluid or air from an organ or cavity by needle
9. Common name for castrating a horse
11. Medical term for withdrawal of fluid or air from an organ or cavity by needle
13. Prefix referring to pus
14. Study of tumors or cancer
17. One who studies or treats diseases of the nervous system
19. A nurse or technician trained to administer anesthesia
22. Flushing of the rectum with fluid
23. One who studies or treats diseases of the urinary system
24. Diagnosis by light tapping blows
25. To surgically remove tissue or part of an organ

Down

1. Medical science using irradiation (x-rays)
2. To place a tube into the trachea or stomach via the mouth or nose
3. Study of reproduction and reproductive disorders in animals
5. What a hematologist studies
7. Study of poisons
8. Doctor of Philosophy
10. Common name for tail amputation
11. Diagnosis by feeling with the hands and fingers
12. Indications of disease in a patient
15. Adjective pertaining to a problem caused by medical personnel
16. Study of disorders of the very young
18. Common term for surgical sterilization of an animal
20. Common term for ovariohysterectomy
21. To file off the sharp points on a horse's teeth

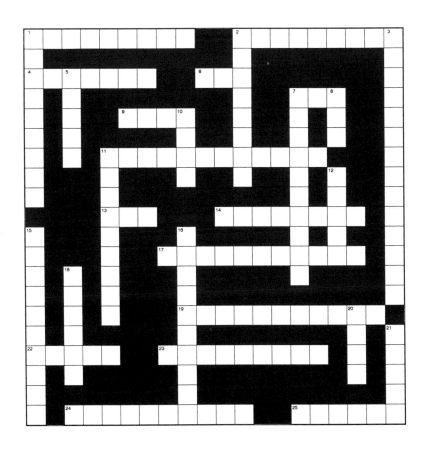

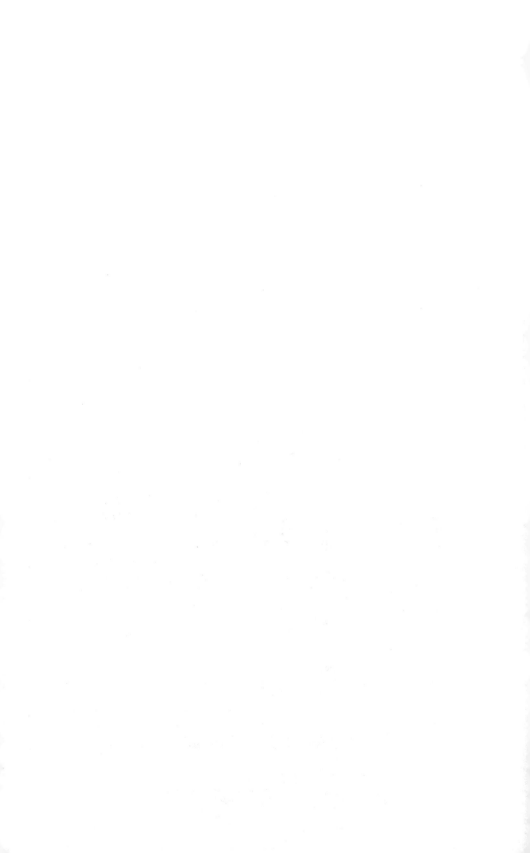

Lesson 7

Important Medical Prefixes

Table 1 contains some important medical prefixes related to disease or pathologic processes. As mentioned in Lesson 3, prefixes can also be expressed in a combining form ("/o"). That is, the "o" is used as a combining vowel.

Table 1. Some important prefixes relating to disease.

Prefix	Meaning	Example and Definition
ANkyl/o	bent, looped, fused	ANkyLOsis: stiffening or immobility of a joint
CRYPt/o	hidden, concealed, depression on a surface	crypTORchidism: lack of testicular descent into the scrotum
LIth/o	stone, calculus	lithlasis: presence of stones or calculi in a hollow organ
MEGal/o MEGa-	abnormally large enlarged	MEGacolon: an enlarged or dilated colon
NECr/o	dead, decaying	neCROsis: condition characterized by dead or dying tissues
PHAG/o	eating, swallowing	PHAGocyte: cell capable of consuming other cells or foreign substances
scler/o	hardening	scleROsis: condition characterized by hardened tissue
THERm/o	relating to heat	therMOMeter: device for measuring body temperature

Note: Throughout this book, syllables with a primary (greater) accent are printed in **BOLDFACED CAPITAL LETTERS**, while syllables with a secondary (lesser) accent are printed in CAPITAL LETTERS only. Unaccented syllables are printed in small letters

(Table 1 continued)

Prefix	Meaning	Example and Definition
THROMb/o	clot	thromBOsis: condition in which a clot forms in a blood vessel
trauma-, trauMAto-	wound, injury	trauMAtic: caused by a wound or injury
TOX/o, TOXi-, TOXic/o	toxins, poisons	TOXiCOLogy: study of toxins and poisons

Table 2 contains some important medical suffixes related to disease or pathologic processes.

Table 2. Some important suffixes relating to disease.

Suffix	Meaning	Example and Definition
-lith	stone, calculus	Urolith: calculus in the urinary tract
-LYsis	destruction of	OSteOLysis: destruction of bone
-maLAcia	softening	MYelomaLAcia: softening of the spinal cord
-MEGaly	abnormally large, enlarged	CARdioMEGaly: an enlarged heart
-paREsis	weakness, slight or partial paralysis	HEMipaREsis: weakness on one side of the body, caused by neurologic dysfunction
-PHAGIa	eating, swallowing	dysPHAgia: impaired eating or swallowing
-PLAsia	development, relating to cell numbers	HYperPLAsia: condition characterized by an abnormally high number of normal cells
-PLEgia	paralysis	HEMiPLEgia: paralysis of one side of the body
-pnea	breathing	DYSPnea: impaired or labored breathing
-RRHEXis	rupture	ANgioRRHEXis: rupture of a vessel
-RRHEa	flow or discharge	DIaRRHEa: abnormally frequent defecation or liquid feces
-THERmia,	relating to heat	HYperTHERmia: abnormally high body temperature

(Table 2 continued)

Prefix	Meaning	Example and Definition
-trophy	relating to nutrition or nourishment, cell size	hyPERtrophy: organ enlargement through increased size of constituent cells
-spasm	twitching, abnormal tractions of muscles	BRONchospasm: spasmodic contraction of the bronchi
-STAsis	stable, constant level	HEmoSTAsis: arrest of bleeding
TOXin	poison	**NEPH**roTOXin: substance that destroys kidney cells

Word Drill A

Using the definitions below, fill in the blank spaces with the correct medical word using the word construction techniques you have learned. The correct answers are listed in Appendix 1.

1. Toxin that kills tissues: _____

2. Abnormally small eyes: _____

3. Softening of bone: _____

4. Stone or calculus in the kidney: _____

5. State of not breathing: _____

6. Enlarged liver: _____

7. Enlarged or dilated esophagus: _____

8. Dissolution of a stone or calculus: _____

9. Hardening and inflammation of the skin: _____

10. Spasm of the larynx: _____

11. Impaired nourishment of cells: _____

12. Enlarged spleen: _____

13. Loving or preferring heat: _____

14. Fear of eating: _____

15. Paralysis in all 4 limbs (hint: use *quadri-* or *tetra-* ,
meaning 4, as the prefix):_____

16. Weakness or partial paralysis of the rear legs (hint: use
para-, meaning beside, as the prefix): _____

17. Incomplete development of an organ because of
insufficient cells: _____

18. Complete cessation of eating: _____

19. Rupture of an artery: _____

20. Discharge of pus:_____

21. Study of disorders caused by trauma: _____

22. Destruction of a thrombus or clot:_____

23. Cessation of contractions of the intestines: _____

_____

24. Abnormally low body temperature: _____

25. Abnormally rapid respiration: _____

Word Drill B: Important Words

Following are words related to diseases or pathologic processes. These words cannot be defined by word analysis. Try to
define each word, then look up the phonetic spelling and definition in the glossary (Appendix 2). Write the correct phonetic
spellings and definitions in the spaces provided.

1. abscess: _____

_____

2. adhesion:_____

_____

3. anomaly: _____

_____

4. ascites:_____

_____

5. benign: _____

_____

6. cancer: _____

_____

7. congenital: _____

_____

8. edema: _____

_____

9. embolism: _____

_____

10. fistula: _____

_____

11. friable: _____

_____

12. granulation: _____

_____

13. icterus: _____

_____

14. jaundice: _____

_____

15. lesion: _____

_____

16. metastasis: _____

_____

17. neoplasm: _____

_____

18. prolapse: _____

_____

19. purulent: _____

_____

20. putrefaction:_____

_____

21. remission: _____

_____

22. rigor mortis: _____

_____

23. tamponade:_____

_____

24. thrombus: _____

_____

25. tumor: _____

_____

Word Drill C

Using the clues provided on the following page, fill in the appropriate boxes. The correct answers are listed in Appendix 1.

Across

. Growth by increase in cell size
. Inflammation of a muscle
. Swelling caused by fluid in the intercellular spaces
. Not malignant
. Softening of the spinal cord
. Spread of cancer cells
7. Death of tissue
2. Suffix meaning weakness
4. Animal with retained testicles
5. Combining form for difficult, painful or abnormal
6. Plural ending for words ending in "-is"
8. Incomplete development of an organ
9. Combining form for the urinary tract or urine
0. Enlargement of the colon
1. Draining tract

Down

1. Weakness on one side of the body
2. Suffix for a cutting instrument
4. Poisonous substance
5. Cessation of breathing
7. Abnormal or diseased area of tissue
8. The stiffening of a joint
9. Suffix meaning paralysis
10. Condition characterized by calculi in the urinary tract
12. Of rapid onset
15. Hardening of tissue
16. Stoppage of bleeding
18. Impaired breathing
19. Yellowing of tissues by bile salts
20. Top or point of an organ
21. Plural for the center of a pathologic process
23. Liquid feces
27. Body part for the combining form ocul/o

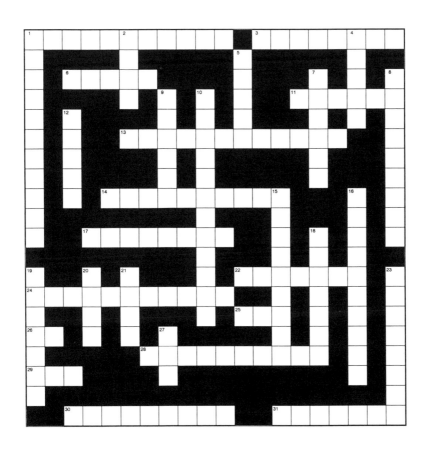

Lesson 8

Terms for Direction, Position and Movement

Following is a list of words used in veterinary terminology to describe direction or position relative to other body parts. Figures 1-3 illustrate these directional and positional terms as applied to people and animals.

AnTErior: pertaining to the front of the body, or denoting a position more forward or toward the front of the body than some other body part. In veterinary medicine its use is restricted to some parts of the head and eye. In human medicine it pertains to the front surface of the erect body. For example, the front of a person's leg is the anterior aspect of the leg.

PosTErior: pertaining to the rear of the body, or denoting a position more toward the rear of the body than some other body part. In veterinary medicine its use is restricted to some parts of the head and eye. In human medicine it pertains to the back surface of the erect body. For example, the back or rear of a person's leg is the posterior aspect of the leg.

CRAnial: pertaining to the cranium or head end of the body, or denoting a position more toward the cranium or head end

---

Note: Throughout this book, syllables with a primary (greater) accent are printed in **BOLDFACED CAPITAL LETTERS,**, while syllables with a secondary (lesser) accent are printed in CAPITAL LETTERS only. Unaccented syllables are printed in small letters.

of the body than some other body part. For example, the shoulder is cranial to the tail (Fig 1).

CAUdal: pertaining to the tail end of the body, or denoting a position more toward the tail or rear of the body than some other body part. For example, the hip is caudal to the head (Fig 1).

CePHALic: pertaining to the head end of the body. This term is not used as often in veterinary medicine as the term cranial. For example, a person's ear is cephalic to the knee.

ROStral: pertaining to the nose end of the head or body, or toward the nose. For example, the nose is rostral to the eyes (Fig 1).

DORsal: pertaining to the back area (topline) of quadrupeds (animals with 4 legs), or denoting a position more toward the back than some other body part. For example, the spine is dorsal to the abdomen (Fig 1).

VENtral: pertaining to the underside of quadrupeds, or denoting a position more toward the underside than some other body part. For example, the intestines are ventral to the spine (Fig 1).

MEdial: denoting a position closer to the median plane of the body or a structure, toward the middle or median plane (see "median plane" below), or pertaining to the middle or a position closer to the median plane of the body or a structure. For example, the medial surface of the leg is the "inside" surface (Fig 1).

LATeral: denoting a position farther from the median plane (see "median plane" below) of the body or a structure, on or toward the side away from the median plane, or pertaining to the side of the body or a structure. For example, the lateral surface of the leg is the "outside" surface (Fig 1).

AXial: pertaining to or situated near a longitudinal line about which a body or structure would rotate.

PeRIPHeral: pertaining to or situated near the areas or surfaces of the body or a structure most distant from their origin or central axis. For example, the skin is peripheral to the underlying muscles.

SuPErior: above, directed above, or pertaining to that which is above. In veterinary medicine, its use is restricted to some parts of the head. For example, the nasal canal in a person is superior to the mouth.

InFErior: below, underneath, directed below, or pertaining to that which is below. In veterinary medicine, its use is restricted to some parts of the head. For example, the mouth in a person is inferior to the nasal canal.

Deep: situated far beneath the surface; not superficial. For example, the bones are deep to the skin.

SUperFIcial: near the surface; not deep. For example, the skin is superficial to the underlying bones.

AdJAcent: next to, adjoining, close to. For example, the tongue is adjacent to the teeth.

PROXimal: nearest to the central axis of the body, relative to another body part, or a location on a body part relative to another more distant location. For example, the femur is proximal to the tibia; the proximal humerus is the part nearer the shoulder (Fig 1).

DIStal: farthest from the center of the body, relative to another body part, or a location on a body part relative to another closer location. For example, the tibia is distal to the femur; the distal humerus is the part nearer the radius (Fig 1).

ObLIQUE: on a plane not parallel to 1 of the 3 major directional axes (medial-lateral, dorsal-ventral, cranial-caudal). For example, the vein crossed obliquely from the dorsal left side to the ventral right side.

MEdian plane: plane dividing the body into equal left and right halves (Fig 1). This is also called a midSAGittal plane.

SAGittal plane (also called PARaMEdian plane): plane parallel to the median plane, dividing the body into unequal right and left portions (Fig 1).

Figure 1. Terms denoting position in animals. (From *Textbook of Veterinary Anatomy,* K.M. Dyce *et al,* courtesy of W.B. Saunders)

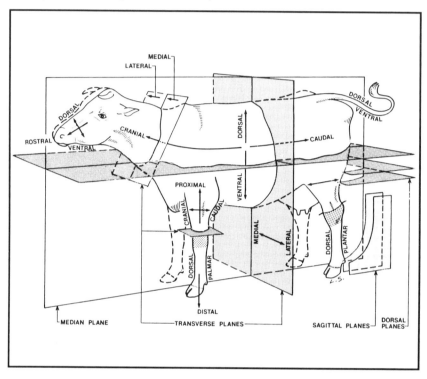

Trans**VERSE** plane (also called FRONtal plane): plane dividing the body into cranial and caudal portions, not necessarily of equal size.

DORsal plane: plane dividing the body into dorsal and ventral portions, not necessarily equal, and oriented at right angles to the median plane (Fig 1).

QUADrants: 1 of 4 parts. For example, the abdominal cavity is traditionally divided into quadrants using the midabdominal transverse and median planes as the dividing lines.

ReCUMbent: lying down. Addition of a modifying term describes the body surface on which the animal is lying. For example, dorsal recumbency means the animal is lying on its back, with the abdomen up.

SUpine: in dorsal recumbency. SUpiNAtion is the act of turning the body or leg so its ventral aspect is up.

Prone: in ventral recumbency. ProNAtion is the act of turning the body or leg so its ventral aspect is down.

PALmar (also called VOlar): the caudal surface of the front foot distal to the antebrachiocarpal joint; the undersurface of the front foot (Fig 1).

PLANtar: the caudal surface of the back foot distal to the tarsocrural joint; the undersurface of the rear foot (Fig 1).

AbDUCtion: movement of a limb away from the median plane of the body (Fig 2).

AdDUCtion: movement of a limb toward the median plane of the body (Fig 2).

RoTAtion: turning about an axis.

EVERsion: turning inside out.

FLEXion: bending. For example, flexion of a joint (Fig 3).

Table 1. Some standardized terms used to denote body position or direction. (From *Veterinary Radiology* 26:2-9, 1985)

Head	Neck, Trunk, Tail	Limbs
rostrodorsal	craniodorsal	cranioproximal
rostroventral	cranioventral	craniodistal
caudodorsal	caudodorsal	craniomedial
caudoventral	caudoventral	craniolateral
dorsomedial		caudoproximal
ventromedial		caudodistal
dorsolateral		caudomedial
ventrolateral		caudolateral
		dorsoproximal
		dorsodistal
		dorsomedial
		dorsolateral
		(plantaro)palmaroproximal
		(plantaro)palmaroproximal
		(plantaro)palmaromedial
		(plantaro)palmarolateral

Figure 2. Terms denoting limb movement: adduction and abduction. (From *Anatomy and Physiology of Farm Animals*, courtesy of Lea & Febiger)

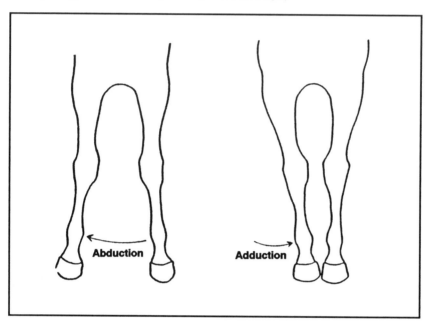

ExTENsion: straightening, such as a joint, or movement by which component parts are pulled apart to lengthen the whole part. For example, extension of the leg (Fig 3).

These terms are often combined to accurately indicate direction or position of a body part. Table 1 lists the preferred combinations used for this purpose.

In radiography these terms are often combined to describe an animal's position relative to an x-ray beam entering and exiting the body. For example, an animal placed on an x-ray table in dorsal recumbency is in the ventral-dorsal or ventrodorsal position because the x-rays enter the ventral aspect of the body and exit the dorsal aspect. Radiography of the legs of animals uses a number of terms interchangeably. For example, x-rays penetrating a front leg or foot from front (cranial or dorsal) to back (caudal or palmar) would produce a dorsopalmar or craniocaudal radiograph (Fig 1).

Figure 3. Terms denoting limb movement: flexion and extension. (From *Anatomy and Physiology of Farm Animals*, courtesy of Lea & Febiger)

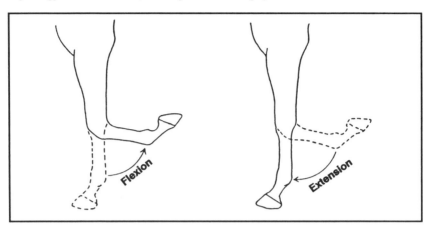

Positional Terms Pertaining to the Teeth

Table 2 lists positional terms relating to the teeth. These terms are also illustrated in Figure 4.

Prefixes for Direction, Position and Movement

Table 3 lists prefixes for direction, position and movement.

Table 2. Positional terms relating to the teeth.

oCCLUsal: surface of a caudal tooth that contacts the opposing tooth when the jaws are closed; the chewing or biting surface. As a directional term, it means toward the chewing or biting surface.

BUCCal: surface of a caudal tooth facing the cheek. As a directional term, it means toward the cheek.

LINgual: surface of a tooth facing the tongue. As an adjective, it pertains to the tongue.

CONtact: surface of a tooth in contact with the next tooth in the same row.

DIStal: contact surface of a tooth, farthest from the midline of the dental arcade.

MEsial:contact surface of a tooth, closest to the midline of the dental arcade.

Figure 4. Positional terms pertaining to the teeth. This illustrates teeth in the upper dental arcade, as seen from a ventral view.

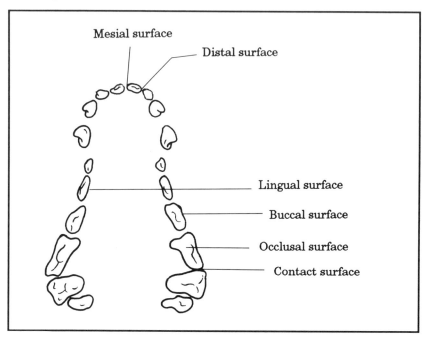

Suffixes for Direction, Position and Movement

Table 4 lists suffixes pertaining to direction, position and movement.

Word Drill A

Fill in the blank spaces with the medical term that best completes the sentence. The correct answers are listed in Appendix 1.

1. The opposite of dorsal is _____.

2. Ventral recumbency is the same as the _____

_____ position.

3. Blood flowing toward the head is moving _____

_____ , and blood flowing toward the tail is

moving _____.

Table 3. Some important prefixes relating to disease.

Prefix	Meaning	Example and Definition
ab-	away from	abDUCtion: movement of a limb or part away from the median plane
ad-	toward	adDUCtion: movement of a limb or part toward the median plane
CIRcum-	around, surrounding	CIRcumanal: surrounding the anus
CONtra-	against, opposed, opposite	CONtraFISSure: fracture in a part opposite to site of a blow
ECt/o	on the outside, outer	ECtoderm: outer germ layer of embryonic tissue
EX/o	outside, outward	EXophTHALmos: abnormal protrusion of the eyeball(s)
ENd/o	inward, inside, within	ENdoCARdium: membrane lining the heart chambers
EPi-	on or upon	EPiDERmis: most superficial layer of the skin
EXtra-	outside of, beyond, in addition	EXtraCELLular: outside of the cell
INfra-	beneath, below	INfraTRAcheal: beneath the trachea
IPsi-	same	IPsiLATeral: situated on the same side
MES/o	middle, intermediate, pertaining to the mesentery	MESoMETRium: portion of the broad ligament suspending the uterus
MEta-, met-	beyond, after, next, change, exchange, transformation	METaCARpal: pertaining to the area distal to the carpus
PARa-	beside, beyond, accessory to, apart from	PARaMEdian: parallel to and beside the median plane
PERI	around	PERiAnal: around the anus
RETro-	backward, behind	RETroPERitoNEal: behind the peritoneum; between the peritoneum and abdominal wall
sub-	under, near, almost, moderately	subNORmal: less than normal
SUpra	above, over	SUpraNAsal: above the nose
trans-	across, through, beyond	transPLANtar: across the sole of the rear foot or hoof

Table 4. Suffixes relating to direction, position and movement.

Suffix	Meaning	Example and Definition
-ad	directed toward, in the direction of	CAUdad(CAUdally): in the direction of the rear or tail end of the body
-um	forms a noun referring to an area of the body	DORsum: vertebral or back area of the body

4. The elbow joint is _____ to the shoulder
   joint but _____ to the front paw.
5. A frontal plane divides the body into _____
   and _____ parts.
6. In medical terms, the "inside" of the leg is the _____
   _____ aspect of the leg.
7. The undersurface of the rear foot or hoof is called the _____
   _____ surface.
8. The act of turning a paw or foreleg so that the palmar
   surface is down is called _____.
9. The heart is _____ to the sternum.
10. The act of moving a leg or part away from the body or
central axis is called _____.

Word Drill B

Using word analysis, define the following medical words
and write their phonetic spellings in the spaces provided. The
correct answers are listed in Appendix 1. The phonetic spellings are located in the glossary (Appendix 2). Remember to
compare your definitions to those in the glossary.

1. contralateral: _____

_____

2. abnormal: _____

_____

3. paravertebral: _____

_____

4. perivascular: _____

_____

5. retrobulbar (hint: bulbar refers to eyeball): _____

_____

6. exoskeleton: _____

_____

7. endocarditis: _____

_____

8. subacute: _____

_____

9. metestrus: _____

_____

10. transplantar: _____

_____

Prefixes for Numeric Terms

Table 5 lists prefixes relating to numeric terms.

Word Drill C

Using word analysis, define the following medical words and write their phonetic spellings in the spaces provided. The correct answers are listed in Appendix 1. Look up their phonetic spellings in the glossary (Appendix 2). Remember to compare your definition to those in the glossary.

1. unilateral: _____

_____

2. bilateral: _____

_____

3. quadriplegia: _____

_____

Table 5. Prefixes pertaining to numeric terms.

Prefix	Meaning	Example and Definition
Uni-	1, single	UniCELLular: one-celled
bi-	2, double, twice, both	BIfurCAtion: fork, division into 2 branches
tri-	3	triMESter: period of 3 months
QUADr- QUADri-	4	QUADruped: having 4 feet; an animal with 4 feet
MULti-	many, much	MULtiCELLular: having many cells
primi-	first	priMIParous: having given birth only once
SEMi-	half, partially	SEMiCOma: stupor from which the patient can be aroused
HEMi-	half, on one side	HEMipaREsis: weakness on one side of the body
AMbi-	both, on both sides	AMbiDEXtrous: ability to use both hands effectively
DEci-	1/10	DEciLIter: 1/10 of a liter; 10^{-1} liter
CENti-	100 or 1/100	CENtiMEter: 1/100 of a meter; 10^{-2} meter
HECto-	100	HECtogram: 100 grams; 10^{2} grams
MILLi-	1000 or 1/1000	MILLiLIter: 1/1000 of a liter; 10^{-3} liter
KILo-	1000	KILogram: 1000 grams; 10^{3} grams
MIcro-	1/1,000,000 (one-millionth)	MIcron: 1/1,000,000 of a meter; 10^{-6} meter
NANo-	1/1,000,000,000 (one-billionth)	NANogram: 1/1,000,000,000 of a gram; 10^{-9} gram
ANG-	1/10,000,000,000 (one-ten-billionth)	ANGstrom: 1/10,000,000,000 of a meter; 10^{-10} meter or 10^{-7} millimeter
MON/o	1, single	MONoNUclear: having a single nucleus
DIPl/o	2, double, twin	DIPlobaCILLi: bacilli occurring in pairs

4. primigravid:_____

_____

5. multifocal: _____

_____

6. trilobectomy: _____

_____

7. semiflexion: _____

_____

8. hemilaminectomy: _____

_____

9. monogastric: _____

_____

10. centigrade (hint: grade means divisions or gradations):____

_____

Word Drill D: Important Words

The following words are common names for different body parts or areas of the body. These generally cannot be defined by word analysis and therefore must be memorized. Try to define each word, then look up the phonetic spelling and definition in the glossary (Appendix 2). Write the correct phonetic spellings and definitions in the spaces provided. Figures 5 and 6 illustrate the common names for body parts in animals.

1. bar: _____

_____

2. breast:_____

_____

3. brisket: _____

_____

4. croup:_____

_____

5. dewlap: _____

_____

6. flank: _____

_____

7. forelock: _____

_____

8. frog: _____

_____

9. gaskin: _____

_____

Figure 5. Common names for body areas on small animals.

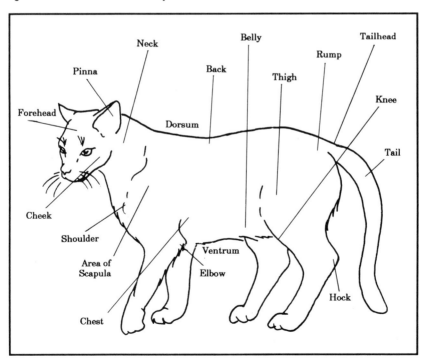

Figure 6. Common names for body areas on horses.

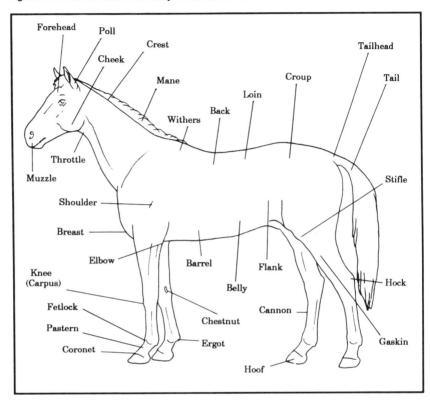

10. loin: _____

_____

11. mane: _____

_____

12. muzzle: _____

_____

13. nape: _____

_____

14. perineum: _____

_____

15. poll: _____

_____

16. rump: _____

_____

17. scruff: _____

_____

18. snout: _____

_____

19. sole: _____

_____

20. thigh: _____

_____

21. throttle: _____

_____

22. wall: _____

_____

23. wattle: _____

_____

24. white line: _____

_____

25. withers: _____

_____

Word Drill E

Using the clues provided on the following page, fill in the appropriate boxes. The correct answers are listed in Appendix 1.

Across

1. Toward the head
5. Lying down
8. Prefix meaning difficult or impaired
9. Prefix for single
10. Toward the back
12. Suffix meaning stone or calculus
13. Chewing surface of a tooth
15. Prefix meaning outside
18. Moving a limb or part toward the midline
22. Prefix meaning 2 or twice
23. Nearer to the center of the body
25. Root word referring to joints
26. Farther from the center of the body
27. Prefix meaning one-billionth
28. To divide into 2 branches
29. Prefix meaning 3
30. Having a single eye or eyepiece
32. Prefix meaning outward
33. Opposite of medial
34. Plural word for the combining form cheil/o
35. Inflammation of the uterus

Down

1. Toward the tail
2. Prefix meaning toward
3. Prefix meaning away from
4. Next to, adjoining
6. Tooth surface adjacent to tooth in the same row
7. Prefix meaning abnormally rapid
11. Prefix meaning under or abnormally low
14. Prefix meaning within
15. Glands that secrete hormones internally
16. Surgery fastening the omentum to other tissue
17. On the opposite side
18. Prefix meaning on both sides
19. Prefix meaning same
20. Situated toward the midline
21. Occurring on both sides
24. Combining form for nose
30. Prefix meaning change or transformation
31. Prefix meaning singular
32. Prefix meaning upon or over

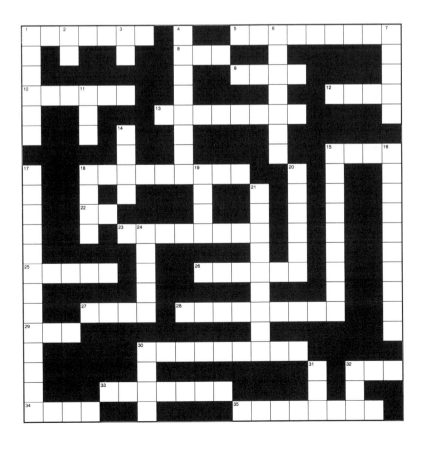

Lesson 9

Terms Relating to Microbiology, Blood and Urine

MICROBIOLOGY

MIcrobiOLogy is the study of MIcroORganisms (microscopic organisms). MIcroORganisms that cause disease are said to be PAthoGENic (patho = disease, genic = to create) and are called PATHogens. Microbiology is divided into the following areas: bacTERiOLogy, the study of bacteria; viROLogy, the study of VIruses; and myCOLogy (myc/o = fungi), the study of FUNgi. PARasiTOLogy, the study of parasites, is a separate discipline not included in microbiology.

Lesson 4 presented the methods of converting singular forms of medical words to their plural forms. The same rules apply to microbiologic terms.

Word Drill A

Fill in the singular or plural forms in the blank spaces below. The correct answers are listed in Appendix 1.

Singular	Plural
1. _____	bacteria

Note: Throughout this book, syllables with a primary (greater) accent are printed in **BOLDFACED CAPITAL LETTERS**, while syllables with a secondary (lesser) accent are printed in CAPITAL LETTERS only. Unaccented syllables are printed in small letters.

---

2. _____   fungi

3. bacillus   _____

4. coccus   _____

5. virus   _____

Nomenclature of Bacteria

Naming Bacteria by Shape

Certain terms are used to describe the shape of bacteria. Listed below are the terms most commonly used.

COCCus: bacterium that is spherical (Fig 1).

BaCILLus: bacterium that is rod shaped (Fig 1).

A bacterium with a shape intermediate between spherical and rod shaped is sometimes described as a coccobacillus.

Some bacteria are named according to their unusual shapes. For example, a spirochete is a spiral bacterium.

Naming Bacteria by Group Arrangement

In addition to terms denoting shape, bacteria are also named for the way they are arranged in groups.

STREPto-: means twisted. These bacteria are found in twisted chains.

STAPHylo-: means bunch or cluster. These bacteria are found in clusters resembling a bunch of grapes.

DIPlo: means pairs. These bacteria are found in pairs.

Naming Bacteria by Shape and Group Arrangement

Bacteria are also named by combining a term describing their shape with a term describing their arrangement. By convention, the term describing the arrangement is listed first when constructing the name of bacteria that occur in groups.

STREPtoCOCCus: spherical bacterium grouped in chains (Fig 1). Example: *Streptococcus equi.*

STAPHyloCOCCus: spherical bacterium grouped in clusters or bunches (Fig 1). Example: *Staphylococcus aureus.*

DIPloCOCCus: spherical bacterium found in pairs (Fig 1). Example: *Diplococcus pneumoniae.*

STREPtobaCILLus: rod-shaped bacterium grouped in twisted chains. Example: *Streptobacillus moniliformis.*

BaCILLus: rod-shaped bacterium grouped in chains that are not twisted (Fig 1). Example: *Bacillus anthracis.*

Figure 1. Shapes and group arrangements of bacteria.

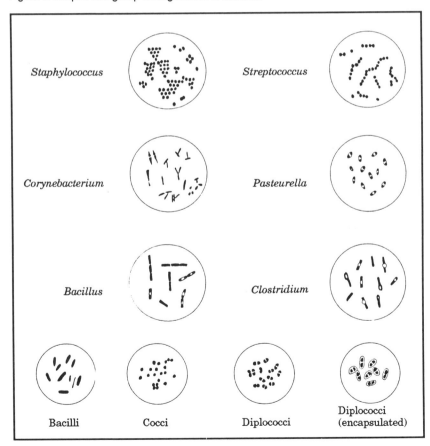

Notice that the genus (first name) is always capitalized and the species (second name) is not, and both genus and species are *italicized*. This is the correct way to write the genus and species for any life form. Often the genus is abbreviated if the species is commonly known, such as *E coli* for *Escherichia coli*, or *Staph aureus* for *Staphylococcus aureus*. If the genus is the main focus of concern and not the species, or if the species has not been identified, it is written as *Streptococcus* sp (a single unidentified species) or *Streptococcus* spp (more than one unidentified species).

Not all organisms are named for their shape or arrangement in groups. Some are named after the person who discovered the organism, or in honor of a famous scientist. Examples are *Escherichia* (for Dr. Escherich) and *Pasteurella* (for Dr. Pasteur). Other names have obscure origins and give no clue as to the organism's shape, arrangement or other characteristics. These names must simply be memorized.

Bacterial Species Names

The species of microorganisms are named by any of 3 methods:
- The species can be named according to the *type of animal it affects*. For example, *Streptococcus equi* affects horses (equines).
- The species can be named according to the *disease it causes*. For example, *Bacillus anthracis* causes anthrax.
- The species can be named according to the *area of the body it affects*. For example, *Staphylococcus epidermidis* affects the epidermal tissues.

Nomenclature of Viruses

Like bacteria, viruses also are named for their shape and other physical characteristics. Others are named for their chemical characteristics or the way in which they replicate. Though viruses may be referred to by their genus and species names, written in italics, it is customary to use their common names. For example, foot-and-mouth disease virus. Following is a list of some comon viruses and a brief explanation of their names.

PoxVIrus (pox-virus): virus that causes pox diseases.

On**COR**naVIrus (onco-rna-virus): an RNA-containing virus that is oncogenic (causes neoplasia or cancer).

Pa**PO**vaVIrus (pa-po-va-virus): virus that can cause *pa*pillomas, *po*liomas and *va*cuolization.

HERpesVIrus (herpes-virus): virus that causes lifelong persistent infections (*herpes* = creeping).

REoVIrus (reo-virus): virus that causes respiratory and enteric infections. The name is derived from *r*espiratory *e*nteric *o*rphan, in that the virus was found in the respiratory and enteric (intestinal) tracts but was not associated with a disease when first isolated (orphan).

Pi**COR**naVIrus (pico-rna-virus): small (pico) RNA-containing virus.

Table 1. Prefixes referring to color.

Prefix	Meaning	Example and Definition
CHLOR/o	green	CHLORophyll: green substance found in some plants that functions in photosynthesis
CHROm/o chroMAT/o	color, colored	CHROmatin: stainable portion of a cell nucleus
cirrh-	yellow-orange	cirRHOsis: chronic degeneration of an organ, often characterized by orange-yellow discoloration
CYan/o	blue	CYaNOsis: blue coloration of mucous membranes caused by poor oxygenation
eRYTHr/o	red	eRYTHrocyte: red blood cell
LEUk/o	white	LEUkocyte: white blood cell
meLAN/o	black	meLANocyte: cell that produces the dark pigment melanin
XANth/o	yellow	XANthocyte: cell containing yellow pigment

Prefixes Related to Color

Table 1 lists prefixes referring to color in biologic, physiologic and pathologic structures or conditions.

Word Drill B

Using the definitions below, fill in the blank spaces with the correct medical word using the word construction techniques you have learned. The correct answers are listed in Appendix 1.

1. A black or dark tumor: _____

2. A single green bacterium: _____

3. Passing of blue urine: _____

4. Abnormal redness of the skin: _____

5. Spherical bacteria occurring in clusters: _____

6. Virus that contains RNA and can cause tumors: _____

_____

7. Rod-shaped bacteria occurring in pairs: _____

8. Toxic substance that kills white blood cells: _____

_____

9. Yellow nodule or tumor: _____

10. Science of colors: _____

TERMS RELATED TO BLOOD AND URINE

Tables 2 and 3 list prefixes and suffixes used in constructing words related to laboratory observations of blood and urine.

Word Drill C

Using word analysis, define the following medical words and write their phonetic spellings in the spaces provided. The correct answers are listed in Appendix 1. Look up the phonetic spellings in the glossary (Appendix 2). Remember to compare your definitions to those in the glossary.

Table 2. Prefixes related to blood and urine observations.

Prefix	Meaning	Example and Definition
cyt/o	cell	CYtoPEnia: deficiency of blood cells
HEm/o	blood, blood cells	HEMorrhage: bleeding
HEma-	blood, blood cells	HEmacyTOMeter: instrument for counting blood cells
heMAt/o	blood, blood cells	HEmaTOLogy: study of blood cells and their disorders
Ur/o	urine, urinary system	Urolith: urinary calculus
Urin/o	urine, urinary system	UrinALysis: analysis of urine

Table 3. Suffixes related to blood and urine observations.

Suffix	Meaning	Example and Definition
-cyte	cell	LEUkocyte: a white blood cell
-cyTOsis	increase in numbers of blood cells, or characterizing the nucleus of blood cells	LEUkocyTOsis: excessive number of white blood cells
-Emia	blood, blood cells	uREmia: presence of urinary constituents in the blood
-PEnia	deficient	LEUkoPEnia: deficient number of wʰite blood cells
-Uria	urine	HEmaTUria: blood in the urine

1. hemolysis: _____

_____

2. erythrocytosis: _____

_____

3. anemia: _____

_____

4. leukemia: _____

_____

5. hematoma: _____

_____

6. pyuria: _____

_____

7. polyuria: _____

_____

8. urogenital: _____

_____

9. cytopenia: _____

_____

10. hemothorax: _____

_____

Word Drill D: Important Words

The following are medical terms related to hematology, urinalysis, microbiology and other laboratory procedures. These words generally cannot be defined by word analysis. Try to define each word, then look up the phonetic spelling and definition in the glossary (Appendix 2). Write the correct phonetic spellings and definitions in the spaces provided.

1. aberration: _____

_____

2. aerobic: _____

_____

3. agar: _____

_____

4. anaerobic: _____

_____

5. artifact: _____

_____

6. asepsis: _____

_____

7. atypical: _____

_____

8. cast: _____

_____

9. centrifuge: _____

_____

10. culture: _____

_____

11. dermatophyte: _____

_____

12. incubation: _____

_____

13. incubator: _____

_____

14. *in vitro*: _____

_____

15. *in vivo*: _____

_____

16. medium (culture): _____

_____

17. morphology: _____

_____

18. papilloma: _____

_____

19. Petri dish: _____

_____

20. pox: _____

_____

21. sepsis: _____

_____

22. streak: _____

_____

23. turbid: _____

_____

24. urinalysis: _____

_____

25. virulence: _____

_____

Word Drill E

Using the clues provided on the following page, fill in the appropriate boxes. The correct answers are listed in Appendix 1.

Across

. Prefix meaning slow
. Rupturing of red blood cells
. Suffix meaning an increase in cell numbers
. Suffix meaning a deficiency in cell numbers
. Pus in the urine
. Spherical bacterium occurring in chains
. Prefix for green
. Suffix referring to urine
. Prefix for yellow
. Cell that produces dark pigment
. Disease characterized by abnormally high numbers of white blood cells in the bloodstream
. Microorganism that replicates only inside living cells
. Deficiency of red blood cells
. White blood cell with a single nucleus
. Destruction or decomposition

Down

1. Rod-shaped bacterium
3. Nutrient medium for bacterial cultures
7. Spherical bacterium occurring in clusters
8. Prefix meaning red
9. RNA-containing virus that causes cancer
10. Prefix meaning urine
11. Deficient numbers of white blood cells
12. Study of blood cells
14. Combining form for joints
16. Blue discoloration of tissue caused by deficiency of oxygen
17. Blood in the urine
20. Urinary constituents in the blood
22. Plant form that does not contain chlorophyll
24. Plug of cellular, bacterial or other debris found in tubules

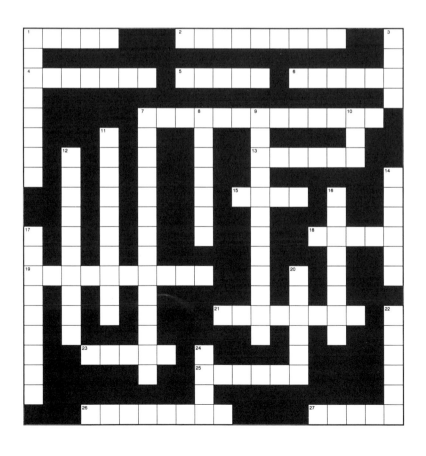

Lesson 10

Other Important Prefixes and Suffixes

Other Important Prefixes

Table 1 contains more of the many prefixes used in veterinary terminology, not covered in earlier lessons.

Table 1. Additional prefixes used in veterinary medicine.

Prefix	Meaning	Example and Definition
ACro-	extremities, top, summit, to an extreme	ACro**MEG**aly: enlargement of the extremities
AER/o	air, gas, oxygen	AERo**PHA**gia: swallowing air
AMbly/o	dull, dim, not clear	AMbly**O**pia: dim vision
aNIS/o	unequal, dissimilar	aNISo**CO**ria: pupils of unequal diameter
ANte	before, in time or place	ANte**FEB**rile: before onset of fever
AUt/o	self	**AU**tograft: transplant of tissue from one part of the body to another
CRYo-	cold, freezing	CRYo**SUR**gery: surgery involving the freezing of tissues
esTHEsi/o	feeling, to sense	esTHEsio**GEN**ic: producing sensation
eu-	good, easy, well	euPH**O**ria: sense of well being

Note: Throuhout this book, syllables with a primary (greater) accent are printed in **BOLDFACED CAPITAL LETTERS**, while syllables with a secondary (lesser) accent are printed in CAPITAL LETTERS only. Unaccented syllables are printed in small letters.

(Table 1 continued)

Prefix	Meaning	Example and Definition
HETer/o	other, another, different	HETero**CHRO**mia: diversity of color
HOmeo-	like, resembling, always the same, unchanging	HOmeo**TRANS**plant: transplant or graft of tisue between individuals of the same species
HOm/o	same	**HO**modont: having teeth of only one type
HYdr/o	water	**HY**drocele: circumscribed collection of fluid
INter-	between	INter**COS**tal: between the ribs
INtra-	within, inside	INtra**VEN**ous: inside a vein
Iso-	equal, alike, same	Iso**THER**mic: having the same temperature
NEo-	new	NEo**GEN**esis: formation of new tissue
noct-,	night, during	nocTUria or nycTUria: frequent
nyct/o	darkness	urination at night
pan	all, entire	PANosteltis: inflammation of all parts of a bone
phon/o	sound, voice	phoNAtion: making sounds or speaking
pre-	before	prePUbertal: before puberty
pro-	before, in front of, in favor of	proLYMphocyte: developmental form of lymphocyte blood cells
post-	after, behind, caudal to	postNAsal: behind the nose
re-	back, again, contrary, replace	reHYdrate: replace lost body fluids
syn-	together, union, in association	SYNosTOsis: union between adjacent bones
toc/o	relating to birth	toCOLogy: study of parturition, obstetrics

Other Important Suffixes and Word Terminations

Table 2 lists important suffixes and word terminations not covered in earlier lessons. Some of these can be used without a root word or another word element. When they stand alone, these words are not hyphenated. For example, esthesia, therapy and tension. They can also be used as word terminations with a prefix to form new medical terms.

Table 2. Additional suffixes and word terminations.

Suffix	Meaning	Example and Definition
-aCOUsia, -aKUsis	to hear	ANaCOUsia or ANaKUsis: deafness, inability to hear
-CAPnia	carbon dioxide	HYperCAPnia: excessive carbon dioxide in the blood
-drome	course, conduction, running	SYNdrome: collection of signs characterizing a disease
-esTHEsia	perception, feeling, sensation	ANesTHEsia: lack of feeling or sensation
-gnos	know, known, knowledge	DIagNOsis: determining the nature of disease
-NAtal	birth	NEoNAtal: newly born
-oid	alike, resembling, similar to	MUcoid: resembling mucus
-Opia	vision	diPLOpia: double vision
-OXia	oxygen	anOXia: lack of oxygen
-para	pregnancy	nulLIPara: female that has never given birth to live offspring
-PHObia	abnormal fear	HYdroPHObia: fear of water
-PHOnia	voice, sound	aPHOnia: inability to make sound or speak
-TENsion	stretching, straining	HYperTENsion: high blood pressure
-THERapy	treatment	CRYoTHERapy: therapeutic use of cold
-TONic	tone, colloidal osmotic pressure	HYperTONic: more concentrated than another solution

Word Drill A

Using word analysis, define the following medical words and write their phonetic spellings in the spaces provided. The correct answers are listed in Appendix 1. Look up the phonetic spellings in the glossary (Appendix 2). Remember to compare your definitions to those in the glossary.

1. prodromal: _____

_____

2. isotonic: _____

_____

3. intramuscular: _____

_____

4. homeostasis: _____

_____

5. hypoxia: _____

_____

6. prognosis: _____

_____

7. dystocia: _____

_____

8. hyperesthesia: _____

_____

9. anisocytosis: _____

_____

10. panleukopenia: _____

_____

Word Drill B

Using the definitions below, fill in the blank spaces with the correct medical word using the word construction techniques you have learned. The correct answers are listed in Appendix 1.

1. Therapeutic use of water: _____

2. Inflammation of the skin on the extremities: _____

   _____

3. Between the digits: _____

4. Before reaching the kidneys: _____

5. After an operative procedure: _____

6. Carcinoma-like: _____

7. Female giving birth for the first time: _____

8. Preferring the opposite sex: _____

9. Excessive fear of darkness: _____

10. Fusion of the eyes into a single one: _____

11. To fracture a bone again: _____

12. Deficiency of carbon dioxide: _____

13. Dimness of vision: _____

14. Fear of sounds: _____

15. Low blood pressure: _____

16. Normal labor or birth: _____

17. Mass or pouch filled with air: _____

18. Without muscle tone or strength: _____

19. Cautery by freezing: _____

20. Toxin produced by the body: _____

Word Drill C: Important Words

The following important medical words have not been defined in previous lessons. Try to define each word, then look up the phonetic spelling and definition in the glossary (Appendix 2). Write the correct phonetic spellings and definitions in the spaces provided.

1. agonal: _____

_____

2. alopecia: _____

_____

3. anorexia: _____

_____

4. antemortem: _____

_____

5. arrest: _____

_____

6. ataxia: _____

_____

7. cachexia: _____

_____

8. colic: _____

_____

9. convulsion: _____

_____

10. emaciation: _____

_____

11. enzootic: _____

_____

12. epilepsy: _____

_____

13. epizootic: _____

_____

14. febrile: _____

_____

15. idiopathic: _____

_____

16. morbidity: _____

_____

17. mortality: _____

_____

18. paroxysm: _____

_____

19. pathognomonic: _____

_____

20. postmortem: _____

_____

21. pruritus:_____

_____

22. pyrexia:_____

_____

23. seizure: _____

_____

24. vital: _____

_____

25. zoonosis:_____

_____

Word Drill D

Using the clues listed on the following page, fill in the appropriate boxes. The correct answers are listed in Appendix 1.

Across

1. Suffix meaning vision
3. Pupils of unequal size
7. Loss of hair
8. Prefix meaning before
9. High blood pressure
13. Insufficient oxygen
15. Prefix relating to the extremities
16. Before birth
17. Prefix meaning the same
22. Female giving birth for the first time
23. Prefix meaning night
25. Stoppage or cessation
26. Collection of signs characterizing a disease
27. Excessive carbon dioxide
28. Between the ribs

Down

2. Deficiency in all types of white blood cells
3. Suffix related to hearing
4. Of equal concentration or osmotic pressure to plasma
5. Feverish
6. Perception, feeling, sensation
10. Prefix meaning good or normal
11. Determining the cause of illness
12. Stage before adulthood
14. Lesion resembling a carcinoma
18. Inflammation of all parts of a bone
19. Difficult parturition
20. Prefix meaning cold
21. Indicating the onset of disease
23. Prefix meaning new
24. Incoordination
26. Prefix meaning together or joined
28. Prefix meaning before

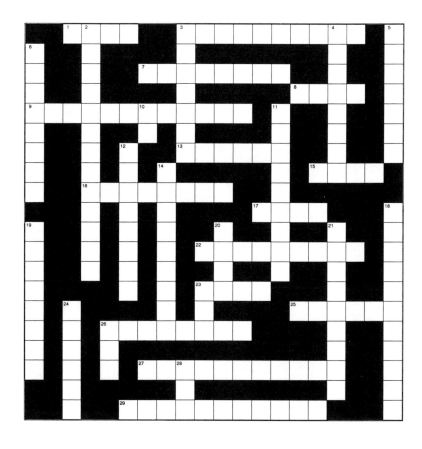

Lesson 11

Terms Relating to Pharmacology

PHARmaCOLogy is the study of drugs and their effect on the body. This science is subdivided into the following areas:

PHARmaCOGnosy: study of the source of drugs.

PHARmacodyNAMics: study of the action and metabolism of drugs and how they are excreted from the body.

THERaPEUtics: study of the treatment of disease with use of drugs.

TOXiCOLogy: study of poisons and other toxic substances.

poSOLogy: study of drug dosages.

A *drug* is a chemical, produced naturally or synthetically, used to treat or prevent ill health. Drugs often have several names and may be available in several formulations (oral liquids, injectables, tablets, capsules, powders, ointments, creams). The word *pharmacy* refers to a retail outlet for the sale and dispensing of drugs, or a part of a hospital (veterinary or human) concerned with preparing and dispensing drugs.

Note: Throughout this book, syllables with a primary (greater) accent are printed in **BOLDFACED CAPITAL LETTERS,** while syllables with a secondary (lesser) accent are printed in CAPITAL LETTERS only. Unaccented syllables are printed in small letters.

Professionals who use drugs for therapeutic means should know as much as possible about the drugs they use; good reference books are therefore necessary.

Reference Books

Excellent reference books on drugs available to veterinarians and physicians include *Veterinary Pharmaceuticals and Biologicals* (VPB) and *Physicians' Desk Reference* (PDR). Other useful references include *PDR for Nonprescription Drugs* and the *PDR for Ophthalmology*. The information provided in the *VPB* and *PDR* is quite similar to the information on the package insert provided by the manufacturer of a drug. Numerous other books cover pharmacologic theory and the different classes of PHARmaCEUticals, grouping drugs according to common effect or mechanism of action rather than discussing them individually. This approach, of course, is very valuable in the study of pharmacology. In the *VPB* and *PDR*, and on drug package inserts, the following information is given: the name (trade, generic and sometimes chemical name); description or composition (what each unit of the drug contains); indications (what it is to be used for); dosage (how much to administer and how often); route of administration (method by which it may be given); side effects (abnormal or adverse effects); contraindications (when not to use the drug); warnings ("Keep out of reach of children"); restrictive caution ("Federal law restricts this drug to use by or on the order of a licensed veterinarian"); and formulation (how the drug is supplied, such as in 50-ml bottles, 7.5-g tubes or bottles containing 250 tablets).

The *VPB* is cross-referenced for convenience when looking up a drug. Drugs are listed alphabetically by trade and generic names (see below), manufacturer and therapeutic use. The *PDR* is virtually the same. The *VPB* also has sections on biologicals (vaccines) for small animals, large animals and poultry, parasiticides, fluids, electrolytes, prescription diets and nutritional supplements, each with its own index. Both books have a product identification section, consisting of color photographs of many tablets, capsules, ointments, vials and liquids.

Appendix 3 lists books available on this topic.

Drug Names

Drugs are named by 3 different methods:

Trade Name

The trade name is the brand name or proPRIetary name. This name usually has the trademark symbol ® or "TM" as a superscript at the end of the name. The first letter of the trade name is commonly capitalized. For example, Amoxi-Tabs®, is a brand name for amoxicillin tablets sold by Beecham Laboratories.

Generic Name

The geNERic name is a chemically descriptive drug name that is not protected by a trademark. For example, amoxicillin.

Chemical Name

The chemical name describes the constituents and their chemical configuration within the drug molecule. For example, D-(-)-alpha-amino-p-benzyl penicillin trihydrate is the chemical name for amoxicillin.

Types of Drugs

Drugs can be classified by their therapeutic use or their actions. Following is a list of some of the most common classes of drugs used in veterinary therapeutics.

ANalGEsics: drugs that relieve pain. For example, aspirin and morphine.

ANesTHETics: drugs that abolish pain, locally or by rendering the patient unconscious. For example, phenobarbital and thiamylal are general anesthetics, while xylocaine and piperocaine are local anesthetics.

ANthel**MIN**tics: drugs that destroy worms. For example, ivermectin.

ANtibi**OT**ics: drugs that inhibit or destroy microorganisms. For example, tetracycline and penicillin.

ANtico**AG**ulants: drugs that inhibit coagulation of blood. For example, heparin.

ANticon**VUL**sants: drugs that prevent or stop convulsions. For example, phenytoin and phenobarbital.

ANtidia**RRHE**als: drugs that combat diarrhea. For example, kaolin and pectin.

ANti**FUN**gals: drugs that inhibit or destroy fungi. For example, griseofulvin.

ANtiin**FLAMM**a**TOR**ies: drugs that decrease inflammation. For example, cortisone is a steroidal antiinflammatory, while phenylbutazone is a nonsteroidal antiinflammatory.

ANtipru**RIT**ics: drugs that control pruritus (itchiness). Many drugs from other categories are also antipruritic, such as antiflammatories, local anesthetics and antihistamines. For example, betamethasone (antiinflammatory), xylocaine (local anesthetic) and promethazine (antihistamine).

ANti**TUSS**ives: drugs that combat coughing. For example, dextromethorphan.

BIo**LOG**icals: drugs of biologic origin, including vaccines, bacterins, toxoids, antitoxins, antivenins and antigens, used to combat or prevent specific diseases or conditions. For example, tetanus toxoid and canine distemper vaccine.

CARdio**VAS**cular drugs: drugs used to treat cardiovascular diseases, such as cardiac arrhythmias, heart failure and hypertension. For example, digoxin.

ca**THAR**tics: drugs that promote evacuation of the bowels (laxatives). For example, dehydrocholic acid and docusate.

ceRUminoLYTics: drugs that dissolve cerumen in the ear (ear wax). For example, triethanolamine.

DIuRETics: drugs that increase urine production. For example, furosemide.

exPECtorants: drugs that promote ejection of mucus or discharges from the respiratory tract. For example, guaifenesin.

HEMaTINics: drugs that increase the oxygen-carrying capacity of the blood. For example, vitamin B$_{12}$.

HORmones: drugs synthetic or derived from animal organs, with an effect on specific organs. For example, oxytocin affects the mammary glands and uterus.

ophTHALmics: drugs used to treat the eyes. For example, gentamicin ophthalmic drops.

Otics: drugs use to treat ears. For example, gentamicin otic drops.

PARaSITics: drugs that control or kill external or internal parasites. For example, carbaryl is an external parasiticide, while praziquantel is an internal parasiticide.

SEDatives and TRANquiLIzers: drugs that reduce excitement and have a calming effect. For example, xylazine is a sedative, while acepromazine is a tranquilizer.

From the above list of drug classifications, you can see that some of their meanings can be determined using the word analysis techniques you have learned. Review the list of drug classifications but do not look at the definitions. Then define each term using word analysis.

Word Drill A

Using word analysis, define the following pharmacologic terms in the blank spaces provided. Also try to provide an example of a drug belonging to each classification. The correct answers are listed in Appendix 1.

1. antihistamine:_____

2. decongestant: _____

_____

3. antipyretic: _____

_____

4. hemostatic: _____

_____

5. antiemetic: _____

_____

Abbreviations Used in Prescription Writing

Table 1 lists abbreviations used for prescription writing and in veterinary records to detail drug use for patients. Because medical records are considered legal documents, it is vitally important that the information contained in the medical records is correctly recorded. It is also important to be able to understand the drug orders written in medical records so that the patient receives the correct dose at the proper interval. As you can well understand, complete comprehension of the following information is absolutely necessary.

Table 1. Abbreviations used in prescription writing and medical records.

Rx:	prescription or recipe	qs:	quantity sufficient
OTC:	over-the-counter		(to provide a certain volume)
	(nonprescription drugs)	po:	per os, by mouth, orally
od:	every day (also, right eye)	ad lib:	as much as desired, or
oh:	every hour		at will
sid:	once a day (not officially	prn:	as needed
	recognized, but often used)	d:	day
bid:	twice a day	c:	with
tid:	3 times a day	w/o:	without
qid:	4 times a day	sig:	write on the label
q:	every	tab, T:	tablet
qd:	every day	cap:	capsule
qh:	every hour	disp:	dispense
q8h:	every 8 hours (substitute	iv:	intravenous
	any number)	im:	intramuscular

Word Drill B

In sentence form, describe the following drug administration orders found in a medical record.

1. Furosemide injection 50 mg/ml, give 2 ml iv q12h.

_____

_____

2. Tetracycline capsules 250 mg, give 1 cap po qid for 7 d.

_____

_____

3. Prednisolone tablets 5 mg, give 1 tab po bid for 5 d,

then 1 tab po od prn. disp. #50._____

_____

Word Drill C

The following terms related to pharmacology generally cannot be defined by word analysis. Try to define each word, then look up the phonetic spelling and definition in the glossary (Appendix 2). Write the correct phonetic spellings and definitions in the spaces provided.

1. allergy: _____

_____

2. antibody: _____

_____

3. antidote:_____

_____

4. antigen: _____

_____

5. antitoxin: _____

_____

6. attenuate: _____

_____

7. bacterin: _____

_____

8. bolus: _____

_____

9. chemotherapy: _____

_____

10. dilation, dilatation: _____

_____

11. diuresis: _____

_____

12. drench: _____

_____

13. efficacy: _____

_____

14. euthanasia: _____

_____

15. fibrillation: _____

_____

16. nebulization: _____

_____

17. parenteral: _____

_____

18. prophylaxis: _____

_____

19. resistance: _____

_____

20. spectrum: _____

_____

21. suppository:_____

_____

22. toxoid:_____

_____

23. transient: _____

_____

24. vaccine:_____

_____

25. vehicle: _____

_____

Word Drill D

Using the clues provided on the following page, fill in the appropriate boxes. The correct answers are listed in Appendix 1.

Across

1. Study of drug dosages
3. Place where drugs are dispensed
6. Abbreviation for 4 times a day
7. Drug that kills fungi
8. Abbreviation for over the counter
10. Abbreviation for tablet
12. Brand or trade name
16. Abbreviation for as needed
17. Abbreviation for intramuscular
19. Abbreviation for every day
21. Drug that alleviates pain or renders unconsciousness
25. Class of drug that is addictive, analgesic and sedative
26. Abbreviation for twice a day
31. Medication for the eye
32. Abbreviation for write on the label
35. Class of drug that combats coughing
37. Effectiveness
38. Body part for the combining form oste/o

Down

1. Study of drugs and their effects
2. Common name for a drug not registered and not chemically descriptive
3. Abbreviation for *Physicians' Desk Reference*
4. Abbreviation for prescription
5. Drug that promotes bowel movement
9. Substance used to treat disease
11. Drug that diminishes pain
13. Per os
14. Abbreviation for 3 times a day
15. Prefix meaning after
18. Group of drugs including vaccines, toxoids and bacterins
20. Abbreviation for Drug Enforcement Administration
22. Abbreviation for intravenous
23. Painless death
24. Drug that increases urine output
27. Substance that stimulates immunity to a pathogen
28. Concentrated mass of a drug given IV at one time
29. Abbreviation for every hour
30. Suffix meaning pain
33. Necessary for life
34. Unofficial abbreviation for once a day
36. Abbreviation for *Veterinary Pharmaceuticals and Biologicals*

Lesson 12

Abbreviations and Symbols

The bulk of this lesson consists of the numerous abbreviations and symbols used in veterinary medicine. Some other pharmacology abbreviations, not covered in Lesson 10, are also presented. It is helpful to know these abbreviations because they are used routinely in veterinary practice, record-keeping, journals, textbooks and seminars. They are also useful as "medical shorthand" for notetaking during class lectures.

Abbreviation	Meaning
AAHA	American Animal Hospital Association
ac	before meals
AHT	Animal Health Technician
AI	artificial insemination
amp	ampule
amt	amount
AP, A-P	anterior-posterior (radiographic position in which x-rays strike the anterior surface of the body part first)
aq	aqueous (water)
ASAP	as soon as possible
ASPCA	American Society for the Prevention of Cruelty to Animals

Note: Throughout this book, syllables with a primary (greater) accent are printed in **BOLDFACED CAPITAL LETTERS**, while syllables with a secondary (lesser) accent are printed in CAPITAL LETTERS only. Unaccented syllables are printed in small letters.

Abbreviation	Meaning
ATP	adenosine triphophate (compound that provides energy for metabolic reactions)
AV	atrioventricular
AVMA	American Veterinary Medical Association
bpm	beats per minute
BUN	blood urea nitrogen
BVD	bovine virus diarrhea
BW	body weight
Bx	biopsy
cal	small calorie (0.001 kilocalorie)
Cal	large calorie (1.0 kilocalorie)
CAV	canine adenovirus
CBC	complete blood count
cc	cubic centimeter (ml)
ccms	clean catch, midstream
CCV	canine coronavirus (vaccine)
CF	complement fixation
ck	check
cm	centimeter
CM	castrated male
CMT	California mastitis test
CNS	central nervous system
CO_2	carbon dioxide
conc	concentration
cont	continue
CPR	cardiopulmonary resuscitation
CPV	canine parvovirus (vaccine)
crit	hematocrit
CSF	cerebrospinal fluid
C-section	cesarean section
CV, CVS	cardiovascular, cardiovascular system
CVT	Certified Veterinary Technician
D5W	5% dextrose in water
DEA	Drug Enforcement Administration
decr	decrease
DES	diethylstilbestrol (an estrogen)
DHIA	Dairy Herd Improvement Association
DHIR	Dairy Herd Improvement Registry
DHLP-P	distemper, hepatitis, leptospirosis, parainfluenza, parvovirus (vaccine)
diff	differential
dil	dilute, diluted
D-M	distemper – measles (vaccine)

Abbreviation	Meaning
DMSO	dimethyl sulfoxide
DNA	deoxyribonucleic acid
DOB	date of birth
dr	dram
DV, D-V	dorsal-ventral (radiographic position in which x-rays strike the dorsum of the animal first)
DVM	Doctor of Veterinary Medicine
Dx	diagnosis
ECG	electrocardiogram
EDTA	ethylenediaminetetraacetic acid
EEE	Eastern equine encephalomyelitis
EEG	electroencephalogram
EFA	essential fatty acids
EM	electron microscope
EMG	electromyogram
eod	every other day (not an official pharmacologic abbreviation, but commonly used)
ER	emergency room
est	estimate
F	female
FAT	fluorescent antibody test
FDA	Food & Drug Administration
fe	female
FeLV	feline leukemia virus
FIA	feline infectious anemia
FIP	feline infectious peritonitis
ft	foot, feet
FUS	feline urologic syndrome
FVRCP	feline viral rhinotracheitis, calicivirus, panleukopenia (vaccine)
Fx	fracture
g	gram
gal	gallon
GI	gastrointestinal
gr	grain
gt	drop
gtt	drops
GU	genitourinary
Hb	hemoglobin
HBC	hit by car
hct	hematocrit (PCV)
H_2O	water
HPF	high-power field
hr, h	hour
HR	heart rate

Abbreviation	Meaning
HS	bedtime
Hx	history
IBR	infectious bovine rhinotracheitis
IC	intracardiac
ICU	intensive care unit
ID	intradermal
Ig	immunoglobulin
IM	intramuscular
incr	increase
inj	injection
IP	intraperitoneal
IPV	infectious pustular vulvovaginitis
KBH	kicked by horse
kg	kilogram; 1000 grams
kVp	kilovolts peak
L	left
L	liter
LA	large animal
lab	laboratory
lat	lateral
lb	pound
LD	lethal dose
LDA	left displaced abomasum
LE	left eye
LI	large intestine
LPF	low-power field
LVT	Licensed Veterinary Technician
M	male
m	meter, mass, milli-
mA	milliamperage
mAS	milliamperage-seconds (product of milliamperage multiplied by seconds)
mcg	microgram; one-millionth of a gram
MCH	mean corpuscular hemoglobin
MCHC	mean corpuscular hemoglobin concentration
MCV	mean corpuscular volume
MDB	minimum data base
mEq	milliequivalent
mg	milligram; one-thousandth of a gram
$MgSO_4$	magnesium sulfate (Epsom salts)
μg	one-millionth of a gram; microgram
μl	one-millionth of a liter; microliter
μ	micron; one-millionth of a meter
min	minute, minum
misc	miscellaneous

Abbreviation	Meaning
ml	milliliter; one-thousandth of a liter
MLV	modified live virus (vaccine)
mm	millimeter; one-thousandth of a meter
mm	mucous membrane
MMA	metritis-mastitis-agalactia syndrome
mo	month, months
MRCVS	Member of the Royal College of Veterinary Surgeons, designation for a licensed graduate of a British veterinary college
NAF	no abnormal findings
NAVTA	North American Veterinary Technicians' Association
nc	no charge
neg (-)	negative
ng	one-billionth of a gram; nanogram
NH_3	ammonia
nm	one-billionth of a meter; nanometer
no	number
NPE, NPx	normal physical exam
NPN	nonprotein nitrogen
NPO	nothing per os, nothing by mouth
NRBC	nucleated red blood cell
NVD	nausea, vomiting, diarrhea
O_2	oxygen
OB	obstetrics
OC	office call
OD	right eye
OD	every day (also qd)
oint	ointment
OL	left eye
OR	operating room
os, ora	mouth
os, ossa	bone
OU	both eyes together or each eye
oz	ounce
P	pulse, pain, procedure
PA, P-A	posterior-anterior (radiographic position in which x-rays strike the posterior side first)
PA	preanesthetic
pc	after meals
PCV	packed cell volume (hematocrit)
pg	pregnant
pg	one-trillionth of a gram; picogram
pH	hydrogen ion concentration of a solution

Abbreviation	Meaning
PMN	polymorphonuclear leukocyte (neutrophil)
POVMR	problem-oriented veterinary medical record
pos (+)	positive
PPLO	pleuropneumonia-like organism
ppb	parts per billion
ppm	parts per million
pr	per rectum
prog	prognosis
PSS	physiologic saline solution
pt	patient
PT	physical therapy
PT	prothrombin time
PTS	put to sleep
PTT	partial thromboplastin time
PU	perineal urethrostomy
pulv	pulverized, powder
Px	physical examination
ql	as much as desired
qn	every night
qs	sufficient quantity
QNS	quantity not sufficient
qv	as much as desired
R	right
R	respiration
RANA	Registered Animal Nursing Auxiliary, the British equivalent of a Licensed Veterinary Technician
rbc	red blood cell
RDA	right displaced abomasum
RE	right eye
REM	rapid eye movement (stage of deep sleep)
RNA	ribonucleic acid
RP	retained placenta
rpm	revolutions per minute
RV	rabies vaccine
Rx	medication, prescription
s, $\bar{s}$, $\dot{s}$, $\underset{\bullet}{s}$, w/o	without
SA	small animal
SA	sinoatrial
SAP	serum alkaline phosphatase
SC	subcutaneous
SF	spayed female
SG, sp gr	specific gravity
SI	small intestine
sl	slight

Abbreviation	Meaning
sm	small
SOAP	subjective objective assessment plan
sol	solution
spec	specimen
SPF	specific pathogen free
sp, spp	species, species (pl)
stat	immediately!
sub-cu, sub-Q, SQ	subcutaneous
Sx	sign, surgery
T	temperature
TAT	tetanus antitoxin
TB	tuberculosis
tbsp	tablespoon
temp	temperature
TGE	transmissible gastroenteritis of pigs
TLC	tender loving care
TMJ	temporomandibular (jaw) joint
TNTC	too numerous to count
TPR	temperature, pulse, respirations
tsp	teaspoon
TT	tetanus toxoid
Tx	treatment
UA, U/A	urinalysis
UGI	upper gastrointestinal (tract)
URI	upper respiratory infection
USP	United States Pharmacopeia
UTI	urinary tract infection
UV	ultraviolet (light)
VD, V-D	ventral-dorsal (radiographic position in which x-rays strike the ventrum first)
VEE	Venezuelan equine encephalomyelitis
VMD	Veterinary Medical Doctor, same as DVM
vol	volume
VT	veterinary technician
wbc	white blood cell
WEE	Western equine encephalomyelitis
wk	week
WMT	Wisconsin mastitis test
wt	weight
yr	year, years

Symbol	Meaning
@	at, each
♂	male
♀	female
+	positive
++++	4 plus positive (can use 2 or 3 also)
−	negative
↑	increase
↓	decrease
<	less than
≤	less than or equal to
>	greater than
≥	greater than or equal to
~	approximately
x	times, for
μ	micron, micro-
✓	check
#	number, pounds
$1°, 2°$	primary, secondary
⊥	proportional, $90°$
α	alpha
β	beta
Δ	delta, change, distilled
γ	gamma
π	pi
$\propto$	proportional to
/	per
≅	equivalent

Word Drill A

In the space provided, write the meaning for the abbreviation given.

1. NPE: _____

2. H_2O: _____

3. DOB: _____

4. VMD: _____

5. 5 gtt/h: _____

6. Neg for FeLV: _____

7. Est 5 NRBC/HPF: _____

8. Place ointment in RE tid x 4 wk: _____

_____

9. On POVMR write Hx, TPR, wt: _____

_____

10. Though NAF on Px, the Dx, based on lab results, was FIP:

_____

11. NAF on D-V and V-D of chest:_____

_____

12. UA showed + + + + protein, SG 1.025, but NAF in sediment:

_____

13. Needs DHLP-P and RV: _____

_____

14. Do TB test by ID inj: _____

_____

15. Cat had Fx of R rear leg after HBC: _____

_____

Word Drill B: Important Words

Following are common words used to describe animals in terms of age and reproductive state. You probably know many common ones. These words cannot be defined by word analysis. Try to define each word, then look up the phonetic spelling and definition in the glossary (Appendix 2). Write the correct phonetic spellings and definitions in the spaces provided.

1. barrow:_____

2. bitch:_____

3. boar: _____

4. brachycephalic:_____

5. buck: _____

6. calf:_____

7. calve: _____

8. capon: _____

9. colt: _____

10. doe:_____

11. dolichocephalic: _____

12. farrow:_____

13. filly: _____

14. foal: _____

15. freshen: _____

16. gelding: _____

17. gilt:_____

18. heifer: _____

19. jack: _____

20. jennet: _____

21. kid: _____

22. lamb: _____

23. nanny: _____

24. queen: _____

25. shoat:_____

26. sow: _____

27. steer: _____

28. tom: _____

29. wether: _____

30. whelp: _____

Word Drill C

Using the clues provided on the following page, fill in the appropriate boxes. Correct answers are listed in Appendix 1.

Across

1. Study of ionizing radiation
6. Referring to the undersurface of the front foot
8. Abbreviation for surgery
9. Degenerative kidney condition
11. Body part for combining form uter/o
13. Common name for tetanus
15. Adult female goat
16. Abbreviation for intradermal
17. Abbreviation for tender loving care
18. Inflammation of the lungs
20. Combining form for rectum
22. Prefix meaning rapid
26. Abbreviation for posterior-anterior radiographic view
27. Abbreviation for Eastern equine encephalomyelitis
30. Abbreviation for one-thousandth of a meter
32. Abnormal rhythm of the heart
35. Abbreviation for feline leukemia virus
36. Abbreviation for one-billionth of a meter
37. Abbreviation for electrocardiogram
39. Top or crown of the head
40. Abbreviation for animal health technician
41. Itchiness
43. Abbreviation for nothing to be given by mouth
44. Abbreviation for immunoglobulin
45. Class of drug that prevents blood coagulation
46. Abbreviation for American Animal Hospital Association

Down

1. Excision of part of an organ or structure
2. Abbreviation for diagnosis
3. Instrument for viewing the interior of the abdomen
4. Abbreviation for urinary tract infection
5. Abbreviation for physical examination
7. Toward the nose or most cranial part of the body
9. Inflammation of the nerves
10. Body part for the combining form splen/o
12. Abbreviation for temporomandibular joint
13. Abbreviation for large intestine
14. Surgically created opening connecting the colon to the body surface
19. Abbreviation meaning immediately
21. Abbreviation for treatment
23. Abbreviation for history
24. Meaning of the abbreviation Hb
25. Blood clot at its site of origin
28. Abbreviation for electron microscope
29. Accumulation of urinary waste products in the blood
31. Castrated male sheep
33. Tumor consisting of darkly pigmented cells
34. Lack of appetite
38. Young female pig
39. Eruptive disease caused by a virus
42. Abbreviation for ribonucleic acid

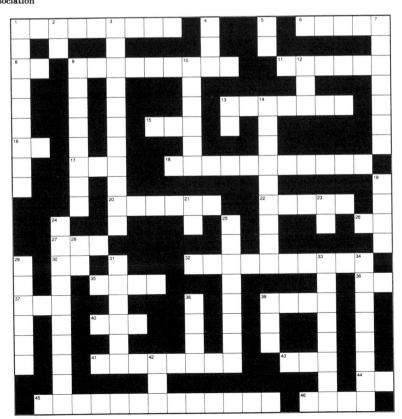

Appendix 1

Answers to Word Drills

LESSON 1

Word Drill A

1. equine surgery
2. canine medicine
3. feline infectious anemia
4. porcine influenza (also swine influenza)
5. ovine leptospirosis
6. pneumonia of rats and mice
7. diarrhea of cattle
8. mastitis of goats
9. beak and feather disease of parrots
10. the cycle of estrus in dogs

Word Drill B

1. ovariectomy
2. ovariohysterectomy
3. hydrotherapy
4. microsurgery
5. carditis
6. hepatitis
7. polyuria
8. cryosurgery
9. microscope
10. dysphagia

(LESSON 1 continued)

11. blepharospasm

12. hoofknife

13. footrot

14. bronchitis

15. polyarthritis

Word Drill C

1. Poly   -   un   -   saturated
   many   reverse of   no double or triple
                                                    bonds between carbon
                                                    atoms
   = many double and triple bonds between carbon atoms

2. Hepato   -   itis
   liver   inflammation
   = inflammation of the liver

3. Horn   -   fly
   horn   dipterous insect
   = a dipterous insect that frequents the area around the horns

4. Blephar   -   itis
   eyelids   inflammation of
   = inflammation of the eyelids

5. Peri   -   card   -   itis
   around   heart   inflammation of
   = inflammation of the area around the heart, specifically
   referring to the sac around the heart

6. Mast   -   ectomy
   mammary(glands)   excision of
   = excision of the mammary gland(s)

7. Poly   -   phagia
   many, much   eating or swallowing
   = eating too much

(LESSON 1 continued)

8. Cryo - therapy
   cold treatment
   = treatment using cold temperatures

9. Arthro - scope
   joints instrument for examining
   = instrument used to examine joints

10. Hemat - uria
    blood urine
    = blood in the urine

Word Drill E

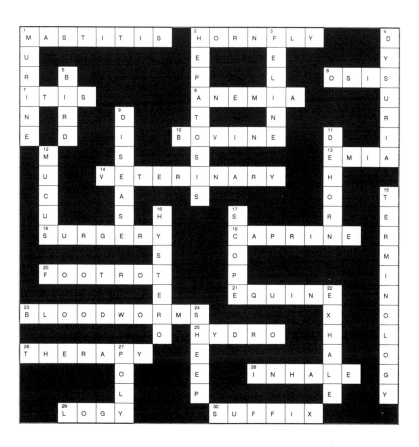

LESSON 2

Word Drill A

1. gastro   -   tomy
   stomach   making an incision
   = incision into the stomach

2. cholecyst   -   ectomy
   gallbladder   to excise
   = excision of the gallbladder

3. abomaso   -   pexy
   abomasum   surgical fixation
   = surgical fixation of the abomasum (to the body wall)

4. rumen   -   ostomy
   rumen   to create an artificial
                        opening to the exterior
   = artificial opening connecting the rumen to the exterior of
   the body

5. pyloro   -   plasty
   pylorus   shaping or surgical
                        formation of
   = surgical repair of the pylorus to improve function

6. gastro   -   jejuno   -   stomy
   stomach   jejunum   to create an artifical
                                         opening between
   = surgically created opening between the stomach and jejunum

7. cholecysto   -   litho   -   tripsy
   gallbladder   stone   crushing
   = crushing gallstones (stones or calculi) in the gallbladder

8. entero   -   tomy
   intestines   to incise
   = incision into the intestines

9. hepato   -   rrhaphy
   liver   to surgically repair
                        by suturing together
   = surgical repair of the liver by suturing (a laceration)

(LESSON 2 continued)

10. rumeno   -   centesis
    rumen   to withdraw fluid
                through a needle
  = withdrawal of rumen fluid with a needle

Word Drill B

1. stomatoplasty

2. esophagotomy

3. splanchnolithotripsy or enterolithotripsy

4. tonsillectomy

5. omasopexy

6. choledochocentesis

7. gastroenterostomy

8. cheiloplasty

9. ileotomy

10. pancreatectomy

Word Drill D

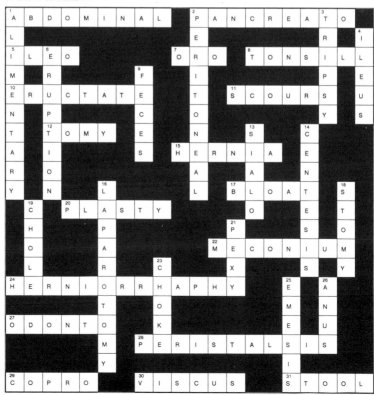

LESSON 3

Word Drill A

1. pyelo   -   nephr   -   itis
   kidney's pelvis   kidney   inflammation of
   = inflammation of the renal (kidney) pelvis and the kidney as a
   whole

2. aort   -   ectasia
   aorta   dilatation (abnormal
              expansion) of
   = dilatation of the aorta

3. broncho   -   pneumon   -   ia
   bronchi   lungs   -   a disease
   = disease of the pulmonary (lung) bronchi.

4. cysto   -   cele
   bladder   hernial sac
   = herniated bladder forming a sac

5. cardio   -   dynia
   heart   pain
   = pain in the heart

6. hepat   -   oma
   liver   tumor
   = tumor of the liver

7. tracheo   -   pathy
   trachea   any disorder or disease
   = any disease of the trachea

8. urethro   -   rrhagia
   urethra   hemorrhage
   = hemorrhage from the urethra

9. uretero   -   py   -   osis
   ureter   pus   abnormal condition
   = pus in the ureter

10. anti   -   diarrhe   -   al
    against   diarrhea   pertaining to or suffix
                       denoting a noun
    = combating diarrhea

11. brady   -   phagia
    slow   eating
    = abnormally slow eating

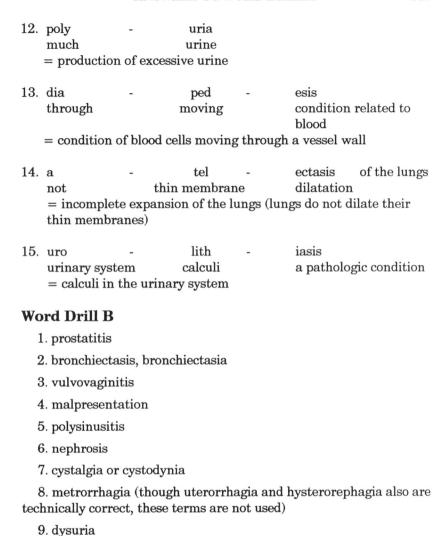

12. poly   -   uria
    much   urine
    = production of excessive urine

13. dia   -   ped   -   esis
    through   moving   condition related to
                                                    blood
    = condition of blood cells moving through a vessel wall

14. a   -   tel   -   ectasis   of the lungs
    not   thin membrane   dilatation
    = incomplete expansion of the lungs (lungs do not dilate their
    thin membranes)

15. uro   -   lith   -   iasis
    urinary system   calculi   a pathologic condition
    = calculi in the urinary system

Word Drill B

1. prostatitis

2. bronchiectasis, bronchiectasia

3. vulvovaginitis

4. malpresentation

5. polysinusitis

6. nephrosis

7. cystalgia or cystodynia

8. metrorrhagia (though uterorrhagia and hysterorephagia also are
technically correct, these terms are not used)

9. dysuria

10. renopathy or nephropathy

11. ascariasis

12. tachypnea

13. pyometritis

14. hyperalgia

15. hypomotility

(LESSON 3 continued)

Word Drill C

1. gastritis
2. tracheotomy
3. pyelolithotripsy
4. splenectomy
5. hepatosis
6. rumenectasia
7. colitis
8. uteropexy
9. orchiectomy
10. dentalgia or odontalgia

Word Drill E

¹L	I	T	H	I	A	S	I	S		²V		³T	H	O	R⁴	A	C⁵	I	C
A										E				M			O
⁶R	R	H	A⁷	G	I	A				N			⁸A	N		⁹P	U	S
Y			L				¹⁰H	E	A	T		¹¹G				U
N			G		¹²M		I				E					L
G			I		¹³C	A	L	C	U	L	U	S		¹⁴I	N	T	A	C	T
O			A		L			A		T		T			T
					¹⁵C	O	N	T	R	A		¹⁶I	A	S	I	S
	¹⁷P	A	T	H¹⁸	Y			I		T		S			O
¹⁹R			Y		²⁰C	H	R	O	N	I	C		²¹A	N	T	I
E		²²H	Y	P	O		N		O			²³P
S		²⁴B		E		²⁵A			N		²⁶D	Y	S		²⁷S
²⁸P	A	R	T	U	R	I	T	I	O	N		O		²⁹N		I
I		A		T		R				³⁰M		T		E		N
R		D		H			³¹B	R	E	E	C	H		P		U
A		Y		³²H	E	A	R	T		T		O		H		S
T				R						R		R		R		I
³³I	N	F	L	A	M	M	A	T	I	O	N		O		³⁴A	B	O	R	T
O				I								X			I
N			³⁵T	A	C	H	Y	C	A	R	D	I	A		³⁶O	S	I	S

LESSON 4

Word Drill A

1. bursae

2. sera

3. nuclei

4. diagnoses

5. appendices

6. carcinomata or carcinomas

7. menisci

8. foramina

9. petechiae

10. specula

Word Drill B

1. atrium

2. datum

3. focus

4. prognosis

5. sarcoma

6. lamina

7. gingiva

8. fornix

9. gyrus

10. syringe, if considering an injection device; or syrinx, if considering a tube or pipe in general or the caudal larynx of birds

Word Drill C

1. spondyl   -   osis
    vertebra   abnormal condition of
    = abnormal condition of the vertebrae (characterized by fusing or ankylosis)

(LESSON 4 continued)

2. parathyroid   -   ectomy
   parathyroid gland   excision of
   = excision of the parathyroid gland

3. lip   -   oma
   fat   tumor
   = tumor of fat cells

4. neuro   -   tripsy
   nerve   crushing
   = crushing of a nerve

5. lamin   -   ectomy
   lamina, flat   excision of
   plate, layer
   = excision of the lamina of the vertebra (flat portion forming the
   tubular structure surrounding the spinal cord)

6. myringo   -   plasty
   eardrum   surgical repair of
   = surgical repair of the eardrum

7. encephal   -   itis
   brain   inflammation of
   = inflammation of brain tissues

8. dermat   -   osis
   skin   abnormal condition of
   = abnormal condition of the skin

9. cranio   -   tomy
   skull   incision into
   = incision into the skull

10. descemeto   -   cele
    Descemet's   sac-like protrusion
    membrane
    = sac-like protrusion of Descemet's membrane (through the
    exterior of the cornea)

Word Drill D

1. pyloromyotomy

2. onychectomy

3. neuropathy

4. meningitis

5. tenosynovitis

6. tibiotarsal joint

7. polyarthritis

8. meniscectomy

9. lymphadenopathy

10. osteomyelitis

11. myositis

12. histopathology

13. keratitis

14. costochondral (junction)

15. lipectomy

Word Drill F

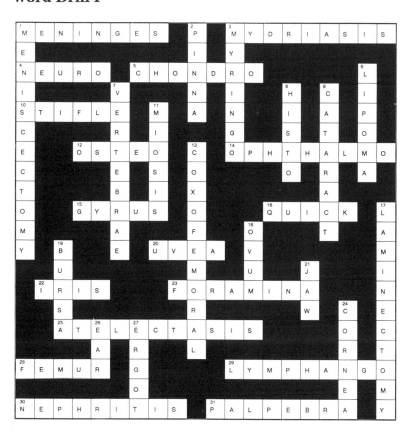

LESSON 5

Word Drill A

1. electro   -   encephalo   -   graphy
   electric   brain   act of recording
   = recording the electrical impulses of the brain

2. echo   -   cardio   -   gram
   reverberation   heart   image produced
   of sound waves
   = image of the heart produced by ultrasonic waves bouncing off
   the heart

3. derma   -   tome
   skin   instrument for cutting
                          thin sections
   = instrument used for cutting thin slices or sections of skin (for
   skin grafts)

4. ophthalmo   -   scope
   eye   instrument for examining
                          or viewing
   = instrument used to view the inside of the eye

5. cysto   -   scopy
   bladder   act of examining
                          with a scope
   = internal examination of the bladder with a scope

6. pelvi   -   metry
   pelvis   act of measuring
   = measurement of the size of the pelvis or pelvic canal

7. arthro   -   scope
   joint   instrument used for
                          viewing
   = instrument used to view the inside of the joint

8. tono   -   meter
   pressure   instrument for measuring
   = instrument used to measure pressures (generally inside the eye)

9. spiro   -   metry
   to breathe   act of measuring
   = measurement of the amount of air moving into and out of lungs
   during respiration

(LESSON 5 continued)

10. gastro   -   scope
     stomach   instrument used for
                         viewing
    = instrument used to view the inside of the stomach

Word Drill B

1. myograph

2. arthroscopy

3. myelogram

4. angiogram

5. microtome

6. mammogram

7. cytometer

8. vaginal speculum

9. colonoscopy

10. bronchoscope

Word Drill D

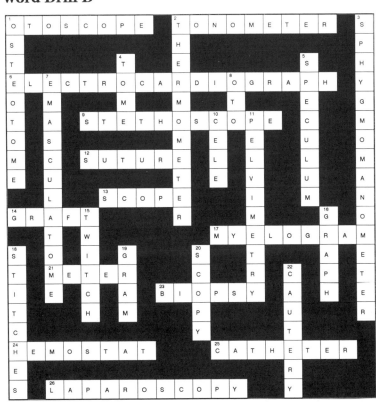

LESSON 6

Word Drill A

  1. urologist

  2. otologist or otorhinolaryngologist

  3. orthopedic surgeon

  4. cardiologist

  5. neurologist

  6. ophthalmologist

  7. dermatologist

  8. theriogenologist, obstetrician

  9. gastroenterologist or internist

  10. toxicologist

Word Drill C

  1. endocrinology

  2. hematology or clinical pathology

  3. lab animal medicine or zoo animal medicine

  4. avian practice

  5. oncology

  6. pathology

  7. neurology

  8. orthopedic surgery

  9. bacteriology, microbiology or clinical pathology

  10. ophthalmology

Word Drill E

Completed crossword grid (row by row):

```
R E S T R A I N T        I N T E R N I S T    T
A                        N                     H
D E B R I D E      C U T                       E
I       L                      T A P           R
O       O    G E L   D    B    T   P   H       I
L       O            O    A        X   D       O
O       D  P A R A C E N T E S I S             G
G       A            K         E   C   S       E
Y       L                          O   I       N
           P Y O         O N C O L O G Y       O
I       A           P              O   N       L
A       T      N E U R O L O G I S T           O
T   N   I           D              Y           G
R   E   O           I                          Y
O   U   N      A N E S T H E T I S T
G   T               T                   P
E N E M A      U R O L O G I S T        A      F
N   R               I                   Y      L
I                   C                          O
C   P E R C U S S I O N        R E S E C T
```

Clue-numbered entries (1 RESTRAINT, 2 INTERNIST, 3 THERRIOLOGY, 4 DEBRIDE, 5 BLOOD, 6 CUT, 7 TAP, 8 PHD, 9 GEL, 10 D, 11 PARACENTESIS, 12 S, 13 PYO, 14 ONCOLOGY, 15 I, 16 P, 17 NEUROLOGIST, 18 N, 19 ANESTHETIST, 20 S, 21 F, 22 ENEMA, 23 UROLOGIST, 24 PERCUSSION, 25 RESECT)

LESSON 7

Word Drill A

1. necrotoxin or histotoxin
2. microphthalmia or microphthalmos
3. osteomalacia
4. nephrolith
5. apnea
6. hepatomegaly
7. megaesophagus
8. litholysis
9. sclerodermatitis
10. laryngospasm
11. dystrophy

(LESSON 7 continued)

12. splenomegaly
13. thermophilic
14. phagophobia
15. quadriplegia or tetraplegia
16. paraparesis
17. hypoplasia
18. aphagia
19. arteriorrhexis
20. pyorrhea
21. traumatology
22. thrombolysis
23. enterostasis (also called ileus)
24. hypothermia
25. hyperpnea

Word Drill C

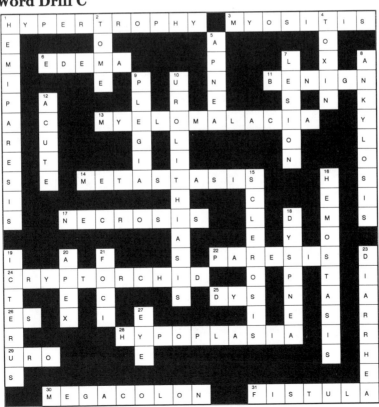

LESSON 8

Word Drill A

1. ventral

2. supine

3. craniad (cranially), caudad (caudally)

4. distal, proximal

5. dorsal, ventral

6. medial

7. plantar

8. pronation

9. dorsal or superior

10. abduction

Word Drill B

1. contra   -   lateral
   opposite   on the side
   = on the opposite side

2. ab   -   normal
   away from   expected or
                         usual
   = not expected or not usual

3. para   -   vertebral
   beside,   pertaining to the spine,
   accessory to
   = beside the vertebral column

4. peri   -   vascular
   around   vessels
   = around the vessels

5. retro   -   bulbar
   behind   globe of the eye (eyeball)
   = behind (caudal to) the eyeball

6. exo   -   skeleton
   outside   support structure
   = support structure located outside the body

7. endo   -   card   -   itis
    inside   heart   inflammation of
    = inflammation of the inside of the heart

8. sub   -   acute
    moderately   occurring rapidly,
                               rapid onset
    = developing moderately rapidly, but not as rapidly as acute

9. met   -   estrus
    next, after   period of sexual
                               receptivity
    = period after the period of sexual receptivity (estrus)

10. trans   -   plantar
    across   pertaining to the undersurface
                               of the rear foot or caudal
                               surface of the rear leg
    = across the bottom of the rear foot or caudal surface of the rear
    leg

Word Drill C

1. uni   -   lateral
    one   side
    = on one side

2. bi   -   lateral
    two   side
    =on 2 or both sides

3. quadri   -   plegia
    four   paralysis
    = paralyzed in all 4 limbs

4. primi   -   gravid
    first   pregnant
    = pregnant for the first time

5. multi   -   focal
    many,   pertaining to foci
    multiple   or centers
    = pertaining to multiple foci or centers

6. tri   -   lob   -   ectomy
    three   lobes   surgical removal
    = removal of 3 lobes (of the lungs or liver)

(LESSON 8 continued)

7. semi   -   flexion
   partially   flexed
   = partially in the flexed position, part way between flexed and
   extended

8. hemi   -   lamin   -   ectomy
   half, on one side   lamina, layer   surgical removal of
   = surgical removal of one-half of the lamina of a vertebra or
   vertebrae

9. mono   -   gastric
   single   pertaining to the stomach
   = pertaining to animals with a single stomach

10. centi   -   grade
    100   gradations
    = something divided into 100 gradations, such as the Celsius
    temperature scale, where 0 degrees is the freezing point of water,
    and 100 degrees is the boiling point of water (at sea level)

Word Drill E

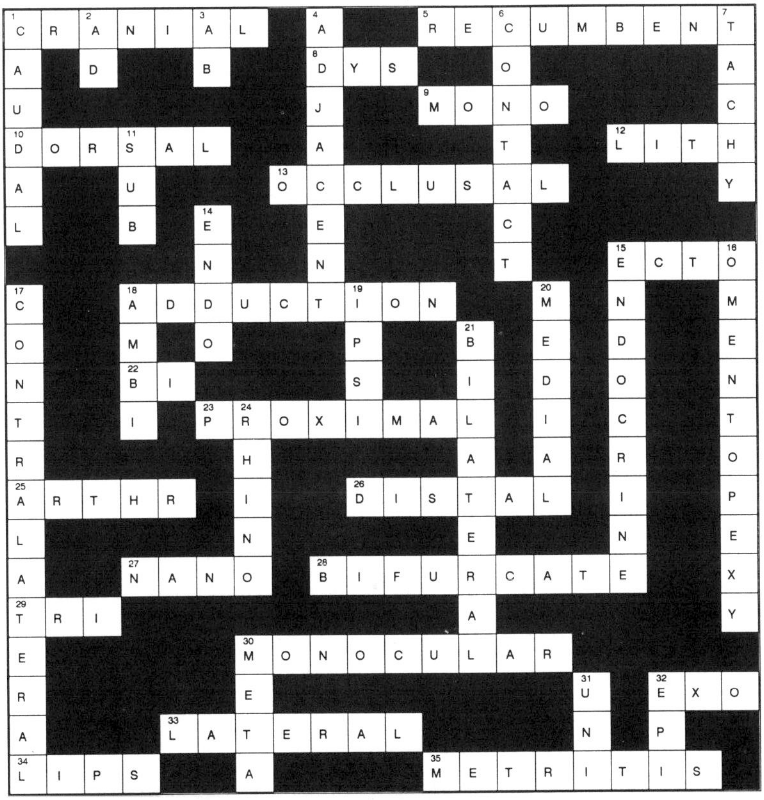

Crossword grid (answers):

```
 1          2         3           4        5        6
[C][R][A][N][I][A][L]   [A]      [R][E][C][U][M][B][E][N][T]
[A]   [D]   [B]      [D][Y][S]      [O]               [A]
[U]                  [J]      [M][O][N][O]            [C]
[D][O][R][S][A][L]   [A]         [T]      [L][I][T][H]
[A]   [U]           [O][C][C][L][U][S][A][L]          [Y]
[L]   [B][E]         [E]         [C]
         [N]         [N]               [E][C][T]      [O]
[C][A][D][D][U][C][T][I][O][N]   [M]   [N]            [M]
[O][M]   [O]         [P]   [B][E][D]                  [E]
[N][B][I]            [S]   [I][D][O]                  [N]
[T][I]   [P][R][O][X][I][M][A][L][I]                  [T]
[R]      [H]               [A][A][R][O]
[A][R][T][H][R][I]   [D][I][S][T][A][L][I]            [P]
[L]      [N]         [E]            [N][E]
[A]   [N][A][N][O]   [B][I][F][U][R][C][A][T][E]      [X]
[T][R][I]                  [A]                        [Y]
[E]                  [M][O][N][O][C][U][L][A][R]
[R]                  [E]                  [U]   [E][X][O]
[A]      [L][A][T][E][R][A][L]            [N]   [P]
[L][I][P][S]         [A]   [M][E][T][R][I][T][I][S]
```

LESSON 9

Word Drill A

1. bacterium
2. fungus
3. bacilli
4. cocci
5. viruses

Word Drill B

1. melanoma
2. chlorobacterium
3. cyanuria
4. erythroderma
5. staphylococci
6. oncornavirus
7. diplobacilli
8. leukotoxin
9. xanthoma
10. chromatology

Word Drill C

1. hemo   -   lysis
    blood cells   rupture
    = rupture of blood cells (generally refers to red blood cells)

2. erythro   -   cytosis
    red   increased cell numbers
    = increased red blood cell numbers

3. an   -   emia
    without   blood, blood cells
    = deficiency in blood, blood cells or hemoglobin

4. leuk   -   emia
    white   blood, blood cells
    = disease characterized by an abnormally high number of white
    blood cells in the blood

(LESSON 9 continued)

5. hemat   -   oma
    blood   tumor, growth
    = growth or tumor-like swelling filled with blood

6. py   -   uria
    pus   urine
    = pus in the urine

7. poly   -   uria
    much, many   urine
    = excessive production of urine

8. uro   -   genital
    urinary   pertaining to the genital
    system   or reproductive organs
    = pertaining to the urinary and genital systems

9. cyto   -   penia
    cells   insufficient
    = insufficient number of cells

10. hemo   -   thorax
    blood   chest cavity
    = blood in the chest cavity or pleural cavity

Word Drill E

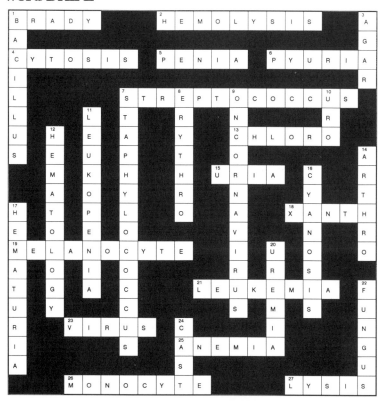

LESSON 10

Word Drill A

1. pro   -   drom   -   al
   before   course   pertaining to
   = pertaining to the time before a condition becomes evident

2. iso   -   tonic
   equal, the   osmotic pressure or
   same as   concentration
   = the same osmotic pressure as that of another fluid

3. intra   -   muscular
   inside   muscle
   = inside a muscle

4. homeo   -   stasis
   unchanging   stabilize
   = unchanging, stabilized physiologic condition of the body

5. hyp(o)   -   oxia
   too little   oxygen
   = insufficient oxygen in the tissues of the body

6. pro   -   gnos   -   (os) is
   before   knowledge   condition of
   = predicted outcome of a disease

7. dys   -   toc   -   ia
   difficult   birth   condition
   = difficulty in giving birth

8. hyper   -   esthesia
   excessive   sensation
   = extreme sensitivity of the senses, especially to painful stimuli

9. aniso   -   cytosis
   unequal   increased number of cells
   = increased number of cells of unequal size

10. pan   -   leuko   -   penia
    all   white   insufficient cells
    = insufficient numbers of all types of white blood cells

Word Drill B

1. hydrotherapy
2. acrodermatitis
3. interdigital
4. prerenal
5. postoperative
6. carcinoid
7. primipara
8. heterosexual
9. nyctophobia
10. synophthalmia
11. refracture

12. hypocapnia
13. amblyopia
14. phonophobia
15. hypotension
16. eutocia
17. aerocele
18. atonic
19. cryocautery
20. autotoxin

Word Drill D

1 O	2 P	I	A		3 A	N	I	S	O	C	O	R	4 I	A	5 F
6 E		A			C							S			E
S		N	7 A	L	O	P	E	C	I	A		O			B
T		L			U				8 A	N	T	E			R
9 H	Y	P	E	R	10 T	E	N	S	I	O	N	11 D		O		I
E		U		U		I			I		N		L
S		K	12 P		13 A	N	O	X	I	A		I		E
I		O	R		14 C				G	15 A	C	R	O
A	16 P	R	E	N	A	T	A	L		N
	E	A		R			17 H	O	M	O	18 P
19 D		N		D	C		20 C		S		21 P	A
Y		I		U	I	22 P	R	I	M	I	P	A	R	A	N
S		A		L	N	Y		S		O	O
T			T	O	23 N	O	C	T		D	S
O	24 A		I		E			25 A	R	R	E	S	T
C	T	26 S	Y	N	D	R	O	M	E	O	E
I	A	Y					M	I
A	X	N	27 H	Y	28 P	E	R	C	A	P	N	I	A	T
	I		R				L	I
	A	29 I	N	T	E	R	C	O	S	T	A	L	S

LESSON 11

Word Drill A

1. anti   -   histamine
    against   histamine
    = agent that combats the effects of histamine

2. de   -   congestant
    removes   congestion
    = agent that reduces congestion

3. anti   -   pyretic
    against   fever
    = agent that combats fever

4. hemo   -   static
    blood   from stasis, to
                               stabilize, stop
    = agent that combats bleeding

5. anti   -   emetic
    against   emesis, vomiting
    = agent that combats vomiting

Word Drill B

1. Give 2 ml of furosemide injection (50 mg/ml) intravenously every 12 hours.

2. Give 1 250-mg capsule of tetracycline orally 4 times a day for 7 days; dispense 28 capsules.

3. Give 1 5-mg tablet of prednisolone orally twice daily for 5 days, then 1 tablet orally every day as needed; dispense 50 tablets.

Word Drill D

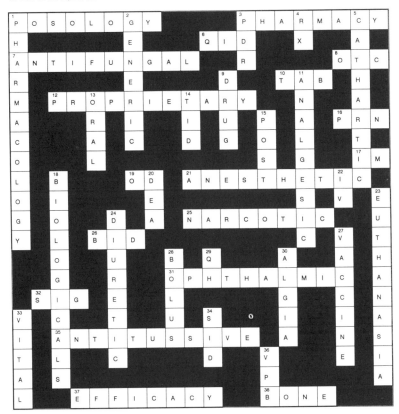

LESSON 12

Word Drill A

1. Normal physical examination (findings).

2. Water.

3. Date of birth.

4. Veterinary Medical Doctor; same as Doctor of Veterinary Medicine.

5. 5 drops per hour.

6. Negative for feline leukemia virus.

7. Estimated 5 nucleated red blood cells per high-power field.

8. Place ointment in the right eye 3 times a day for 4 weeks.

9. On the problem-oriented veterinary medical record, record the history, temperature, pulse and respiratory rates, and weight.

10. Though there were no abnormal findings on physical examination (no abnormal findings), the diagnosis, based on laboratory results, was feline infectious peritonitis.

11. There were no abnormal findings on ventral-dorsal and dorsal-ventral radiographs of the chest.

12. The results of the urinalysis were a 4-plus positive for protein and a specific gravity of 1.025, but there were no abnormal findings in the sediment.

13. The dog requires distemper-hepatitis-leptospirosis-parainfluenza virus-parvovirus and rabies vaccines.

14. Perform tuberculosis test by intradermal injection.

15. A cat sustained a fracture of the right rear leg as a result of being hit by a car.

Word Drill C

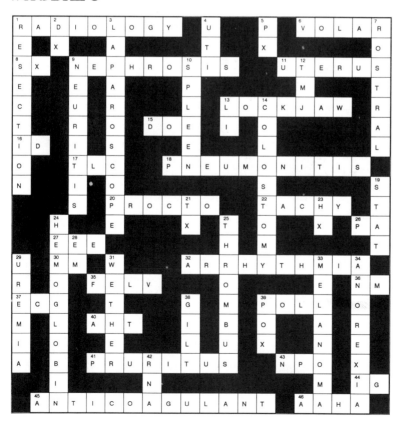

Appendix 2

Glossary

A

a-, an- (ay or ah, an): Prefix meaning without, not having, or the absence of.

ab- (ab): Prefix meaning away from.

abdomen (AB-doh-mehn, ab-DOH-mehn): Portion of the body lying between the thorax and pelvis. Its cavity (the abdominal cavity) contains the peritoneal cavity and its linings and the internal viscera.

abdomin/o (ab-DAH-mi-noh): Combining form for the abdomen.

abdominocentesis (ab-DAH-mi-noh-sehn-**TEE**-sis): Withdrawal of fluid from the abdomen using a needle.

abduction (ab-DUHK-shuhn): Movement of a part, such as a limb, away from the central axis or median plane of the body.

aberration (AB-er-**AY**-shuhn): Deviation from the normal or usual course or condition; imperfection in the refraction or focalization of light, resulting in a poor image.

abnormal (ab-NOR-muul): Not normal; deviation from the usual structure, position, blood values or other physiologic conditions.

abomas/o (AB-oh-**MAY**-soh): Combining form for the abomasum.

abomasopexy (AB-oh-**MAY**-soh-PEHK-see): Surgical fixation of the abomasum to the abdominal wall.

Key to Pronunciation

a=hat • ah=hot • air=hair • al=bell • ay=day • eh=step • ee-deed • er=hurt
eye=fly • i=bit • oh=boa • too=boot • or=for • ow=cow • oy=joy • th=thin
uh=pup • uu=pull • y=fly • yoo=use • zh=measure

---

abomasum (ab-oh-**MAY**-suhm): The true glandular stomach of ruminants.

abort (uh-BORT): To miscarry (give birth prematurely) before the fetus is developed enough to survive on its own; to halt the progress of disease; to halt development.

abscess (AB-sehs): Cavity filled with pus.

acariasis (AK-uh-**RY**-uh-sis): Infestation with mites.

acetabul/o (As-eh-**TAB**-yoo-loh): Combining form for acetabulum.

acetabulum (As-eh-**TAB**-yoo-luhm): Cup-shaped cavity on either side of the pelvis in which the head of the femur articulates.

-acousia (uh-**KOO**-zee-uh): Suffix related to hearing.

acro- (AK-roh): Prefix related to the extremities, top, summit or an extreme.

acrodermatitis (AK-roh-DER-muh-**TY**-tis): Inflammation of the skin of the extremities, specifically the distal extremities and paws.

acromegaly (AK-roh-**MEH**-guh-lee): Condition characterized by enlargement of the extremities, such as the nose, fingers, jaw and toes.

acute (uh-KYOOT): Of sudden onset; having a short course.

ad- (ad): Prefix meaning toward.

-ad (ad): Suffix meaning directed toward or in the direction of the part denoted by the root word to which it is added.

adduction (a-DUHK-shun): Movement of a body part, such as a limb, toward the central axis or median plane of the body.

aden/o (AD-eh-noh): Combining form for a gland or glandular.

adhesion (ad-HEE-zhun): Abnormal fibrous union of tissues; process of joining or sticking together.

adip/o (AD-i-poh): Combining form for adipose tissue or fat.

adipose (AD-i-pohz): Fat; fatty.

adjacent (ad-JAY-sehnt): Next to, close to, adjoining.

adrenal gland (a-DREE-nuul gland): Paired glands lying cranial to the kidneys (one on each side), that produce various hormones, such as epinephrine, cortisol.

adren/o (a-DREE-noh): Combining form for the adrenal gland.

aeluropsis (EE-loo-**RAHP**-sis): Slanting of the palpebral fissure (space between the eyelids), as in cats.

aer/o (AIR-oh): Prefix related to air or oxygen.

aerobic (air-OH-bik): Able to survive only in the presence of molecular oxygen; pertaining to metabolism in which oxygen is involved.

aerocele (AIR-oh-SEEL): Tumor or sac filled with air, often as an outpouching of the larynx or trachea (laryngocele or tracheocele).

aerophagia (AIR-oh-FA-jee-uh): Spasmodic swallowing of air, generally followed by eructation (belching).

Aesculus (ES-kyoo-luhs): Genus of trees, including horse chestnut, containing substances that cause toxicity and bleeding.

affinity (uh-FI-ni-tee): Attraction for, as between molecules, organisms or animals.

afterbirth (AF-ter-berth): The placenta and associated membranes that are expelled from the uterus after the birth of the fetus.

agalactia (AY-guh-**LAK**-tee-uh): Inability, absence of, or failure to produce milk; absence of milk.

agar (A-ger): Mucilaginous substance used to make nutrient media for bacterial cultures and bulk laxatives.

age (ayj): Time elapsed since birth.

agonal (A-goh-nuul): Pertaining to the struggling seen just before death; pertaining to an infection or disease in its terminal stages.

Key to Pronunciation
a=hat • ah=hot • air=hair • al=bell • ay=day • eh=step • ee-deed • er=hurt
eye=fly • i=bit • oh=boa • too=boot • or=for • ow=cow • oy=joy • th=thin
uh=pup • uu=pull • y=fly • yoo=use • zh=measure

ailurophobia (ay-LOO-roh-**FOH**-bee-uh): Pathologic fear of cats.

albinism (AL-bi-nizm): Congenital lack of pigmentation of the skin, eyes and hair. An *albino* is an animal with albinism.

albumin (al-**BYOO**-min): A major protein of blood plasma that is produced in the liver.

albuminuria (AL-byoo-mi-**NOO**-ree-uh): Albumin in the urine.

-algia (AL-jee-uh): Word termination denoting pain or a painful condition.

alimentary (AL-eh-**MEHN**-tuh-ree): Pertaining to food or nutrient, or to the digestive organs.

allergy (AL-ler-jee): Hypersensitivity acquired through exposure to a particular substance (allergen).

allograft (AL-loh-graft): Graft or transplant of tissue between individuals of the same species; homograft, homeotransplant.

alopecia (AL-loh-**PEE**-shee-uh): Loss of hair from an area in which hair is normally present.

alveol/o (al-VEE-oh-loh): Combining form for alveolus, as in the pulmonary alveoli.

alveolus (al-VEE-oh-luhs): A small sac-like structure dilatation; generally refers to the cavity in which a tooth is imbedded, or the terminal sacs in the lungs or mammary glands.

ambi- (AM-bi): Prefix meaning on both sides.

ambidextrous (AM-bi-**DEHK**-struhs): Ability to use both hands in an equally coordinated and effective manner.

ambly/o (AM-blee-oh): Prefix meaning dullness or dimness.

amblyacousia (AM-blee-uh-**KOO**-zee-uh): Dullness of hearing.

amblyopia (AM-blee-**OH**-pee-uh): Dimness of vision without any detectable eye lesions or disease.

ambulate (AM-byoo-layt): To walk.

an-, ana (an, AN-nuh): Prefix meaning up, backward or again.

anabolic (AN-uh-**BAH**-lik): Pertaining to or promoting conversion of compounds into living tissue.

anacousia (A-nuh-**KOO**-see-uh): Total deafness.

anaerobic (A-nair-**OH**-bik): Able to survive only in the absence of oxygen; pertaining to metabolism in which oxygen is not involved.

anakusis (A-nuh-**KOO**-sis): Total deafness.

analgesic (A-nuul-**JEE**-zik): Capable of relieving pain; not sensitive to pain; agent that reduces or eliminates pain but does not cause loss of consciousness.

anastomosis (uh-NAS-toh-**MOH**-sis): Surgical or pathologic formation of a passage between 2 organs; communication between 2 vessels.

anatomy (uh-NA-toh-mee): Study of body structures and their positional relationships to each other.

andr/o (AN-droh): Combining form meaning male.

anemia (uh-NEE-mee-uh): Condition characterized by reduced numbers of red blood cells, and/or reduced hemoglobin.

anesthesia (A-nehs-**THEE**-zee-uh): State of being without sensation, especially to pain. May or may not be accompanied by unconsciousness (general anesthesia vs local anesthesia).

anesthesiologist (A-nehs-THEE-zee-**AHL**-oh-jist): A doctor who specializes in anesthesiology.

anesthesiology (A-nehs-THEE-zee-**AHL**-oh-jee): Study of administration of drugs to induce narcosis and/or analgesia for performing surgery or other procedures.

anesthetic (A-nehs-**THEHT**-ik): Pertaining to, characterized by or producing anesthesia (local or general); agent that produces anesthesia, thus abolishing pain.

anesthetist (uh-**NEHS**-theh-TIST): Person trained to anesthetize patients. In veterinary medicine they are licensed vet-

---

Key to Pronunciation
a=hat • ah=hot • air=hair • al=bell • ay=day • eh=step • ee-deed • er=hurt
eye=fly • i=bit • oh=boa • too=boot • or=for • ow=cow • oy=joy • th=thin
uh=pup • uu=pull • y=fly • yoo=use • zh=measure

erinary technicians. In human medicine they are registered nurses who have attended nurse anesthetist school.

anestrus (an-EHS-truhs): Period of sexual activity between 2 etrous periods.

aneurysm (**AN**-yoo-RIZM): Dilation or outpouching of the wall of an artery, vein or the heart.

angi/o (AN-jee-oh): Combining form for vessel. Usually it refers to a blood vessel, but may also refer to a lymph vessel.

angiogram (**AN**-jee-oh-GRAM): Radiographic image of a blood vessel after injection of a radiopaque dye.

angiorrhexis (AN-jee-oh-**REHK**-sis): Rupture of a vessel

angstrom (ANG-strahm): Unit of measure generally used to measure wavelengths of electromagnetic radiation: equal to 10^{-10} meters (1/10,000,000,000 meter) or 10^{-7} millimeters (1/10,000,000 millimeter).

anis/o (a-NI-soh): Prefix meaning unequal or dissimilar.

anisocoria (AN-eye-soh-**KOH**-ree-uh): Unequal size of the pupils of the eyes.

anisocytosis (a-NI-soh-sy-**TOH**-sis): Increased numbers of red blood cells of unequal size; abnormal variation in the size of red blood cells.

ankyl/o (AN-ki-loh): Prefix meaning stiffening, fusing or bent in the form of a noose or loop.

ankyloblepharon (AN-ki-loh-**BLEHF**-uh-rahn): Adhesion of the opposing edges of the eyelids, fusing the eyelids.

ankylosis (AN-ki-**LOH**-sis): Immobilization and consolidation of a joint as a result of disease, injury or surgery.

an/o (AY-noh): Combining form for anus.

anomaly (uh-NAH-muh-lee): Marked deviation from normal.

anorexia (A-noh-**REHK**-see-uh): Lack of appetite.

anoxia (a-NAHK-see-uh): Absence of oxygen in tissues.

ante- (AN-tee): Prefix meaning before, in time or place.

ante mortem (AN-tee **MOR**-tehm): Before death. When used as an adverb, it is correctly witten as ante mortem. When used as an adjective, it is written antemortem.

antefebrile (AN-tee-**FEE**-bryl): Before the onset of fever.

anterior (an-**TEH**-ree-or): Pertaining to the front of the body, or denoting a position more forward or toward the front of the body than some other reference point or body part. In veterinary medicine it is primarily used in descriptions of the eye.

anthelmintic (AN-thal-**MIN**-tik): Drug destructive to worms.

anti- (AN-ty or AN-ti): Prefix meaning against.

antibiotic (AN-ti-by-**AH**-tik): Substance, produced by microorganisms, capable of inhibiting or killing other microorganisms.

antibody (**AN**-ti-**BAH**-dee): Protein produced by lymphoid tissue in response to exposure to an invading organism or foreign substance.

anticoagulant (AN-ti-koh-**AG**-yoo-luhnt): Agent that prevents clotting of blood.

anticonvulsant (AN-ti-kuhn-**VAHL**-suhnt): Agent that prevents or stops convulsions.

antidiarrheal (AN-ti-DY-uh-**REE**-uul): Agent that combats diarrhea.

antidote (AN-ti-doht): Agent used to counteract poison.

antiemetic (AN-ti-eh-**MEH**-tik): Agent that combats nausea and vomiting.

antifungal (AN-ti-**FUHN**-guul): Agent that inhibits or kills fungi.

antigen (AN-ti-jehn): Any substance that induces an immune response (antibody formation) by the body.

Key to Pronunciation
a=hat • ah=hot • air=hair • al=bell • ay=day • eh=step • ee-deed • er=hurt
eye=fly • i=bit • oh=boa • too=boot • or=for • ow=cow • oy=joy • th=thin
uh=pup • uu=pull • y=fly • yoo=use • zh=measure

antihistamine (AN-ti-**HIS**-tuh-meen): Agent that combats the effects of histamine.

antiinflammatory (AN-ti-in-**FLA**-muh-TOH-ree): Agent that suppresses inflammation.

antipruritic (AN-ti-proo-**RI**-tik): Agent that prevents or reduces itchiness.

antipyretic (AN-ti-py-**REH**-tik): Agent that reduces fever.

antitoxin (AN-ti-**TAHK**-sin): Antibody produced in response to exposure to a toxin produced by microorganisms, insects or plants.

antitussive (AN-ti-**TUH**-siv): Agent that combats coughing.

anus (AY-nuhs): Terminal opening or orifice of the alimentary canal (digestive tract).

aort/o (ay-OR-toh): Combining form for aorta.

aorta (ay-OR-tuh): Main trunk of the arterial system, originating from the left side of the heart.

aortectasia (AY-or-tehk-**TAY**-zee-uh): Dilation (expansion) of the aorta.

aperture (A-per-cher): An opening or orifice.

apex, apices (pl) (AY-pehks, AY-pi-seez): Top, tip or point of a conical organ.

aphagia (uh-FAY-jee-uh): Cessation of eating.

aphonia (uh-**FOH**-nee-uh): Inability to vocalize.

aplasia (uh-PLAY-zee-uh): Lack of development of an organ or tissue.

apnea (AP-nee-uh): Cessation of breathing.

appendage (uh-PEHN-dij): Part attached to the main portion of an organ or the body, such as a limb or ear.

appendix, appendices (pl) (uh-PEHN-diks, uh-PEHN-di-seez): An appendage or accessory organ attached to a main structure. Used alone, it represents a narrow, tubular blind sac at the cecum in people.

appose (uh-POHZ): To place next to or side by side.

arrest (uh-REHST): Cessation of function.

arrhythmia (ay-RITH-mee-uh, uh-RITH-mee-uh): Variation in rhythm of the heart beat.

arteri/o (ahr-TEH-ree-oh): Combining form for artery.

arteriole (ahr-TEH-ree-ohl): Minute vessel branching off of an artery.

arteriorrhexis (ahr-TEH-ree-oh-**REHK**-sis): Rupture of an artery.

artery (**AHR**-teh-ree): Vessel through which blood flows away from the heart to various parts of the body.

arthr/o (AHR-throh): Combining form for joint.

arthritis (ahr-THRY-tis): Inflammation of a joint.

arthroscope (AHR-throh-skohp): Instrument for viewing the inside of a joint.

arthroscopy (ahr-THRAH-skoh-pee): Examination of the interior of a joint with an arthroscope.

arthrosis (ahr-THROH-sis): Joint or articulation between bones; disease involving a joint.

articular (ahr-TI-kyoo-ler): Pertaining to a joint, or to where bones meet.

artifact (AHR-ti-fakt): Any artificial feature, such as that caused by processing of specimens, tissues or radiographs.

ascariasis (AS-kuh-**RY**-uh-sis): Infection by ascarids or roundworms of the genus *Ascaris*.

ascites (uh-SY-teez): Accumulation of serous fluid in the peritoneal cavity from blood vessels or organs.

asepsis (ay-SEHP-sis, uh-SEHP-sis): Lack of infection or contamination by microorganisms.

-asis (AY-sis, UH-sis): Suffix meaning state or condition.

aspirate (A-spi-rayt): To remove fluid or gas from a cavity by suction; to inhale; material withdrawn by aspiration (A-spi-raht).

Key to Pronunciation

a=hat • ah=hot • air=hair • al=bell • ay=day • eh=step • ee-deed • er=hurt
eye=fly • i=bit • oh=boa • too=boot • or=for • ow=cow • oy=joy • th=thin
uh=pup • uu=pull • y=fly • yoo=use • zh=measure

astringent (uh-STRIN-jehnt): Causing local contraction after topical application; agent causing local contraction.

asymptomatic (AY-simp-toh-**MA**-tik): Showing no signs of disease.

ataxia (ay-TAK-see-uh): Muscular incoordination; irregular muscular contraction.

atelectasis (A-teh-**LEHK**-tuh-sis): Incomplete expansion of the lung at birth; collapse of a previously expanded lung.

atonic (ay-TAH-nik): Lacking normal tone or strength.

atrium, atria (pl) (AY-tree-uhm, AY-tree-uh): A chamber. Usually refers to the 2 chambers adjacent to the ventricles of the heart.

atrophy (A-troh-fee): Wasting away of a part.

attenuate (uh-TEHN-yoo-ayt): To weaken; to decrease disease-producing capacity of a pathogenic organism.

atypical (ay-TI-pi-kuul): Unusual; deviating from normal.

auditory (AH-di-tor-ee): Pertaining to hearing.

auscultation (AHS-kuul-**TAY**-shun): Act of listening for sound within the body, usually with a stethoscope.

aut/o (AH-toh): Prefix denoting self, that is, an animal's own body.

autoclave (AH-toh-klayv): Machine that sterilizes medical instruments and materials by use of steam under pressure.

autograft (AH-toh-graft): Piece of tissue moved from one part of the body and implanted on another part of the same body; an autotransplant.

autopsy (AH-tahp-see): Examination of a human body after death.

autotoxin (AH-toh-**TAHK**-sin): Toxic substance produced within the body by tissue changes.

autotransplant (AH-toh-**TRANS**-plant): Piece of tissue moved from one part of the body and implanted on another part of the same body; an autograft.

average (A-ver-ij): Numeric value intermediate between 2 extremes, equal to the sum of all of the values divided by the number of values; mean.

avian (AY-vee-uhn): Pertaining to birds; a bird.

avulsion (ay-VUHL-shuhn, uh-VUHL-shuhn): Pulling away of a part or structure.

axill/o (ak-SI-loh): Combining form for axilla.

axilla (ak-SI-luh); Area ventromedial to the shoulder joint, where the front leg joins the body; the armpit.

azotemia (AY-zoh-**TEE**-mee-uh): Accumulation of nitrogenous urinary wastes in the blood, without apparent clinical signs.

B

bacillus, bacilli (pl) (buh-SI-luhs, buh-SI-ly): A rod-shaped bacterium; bacterium of the genus *Bacillus*.

bacterin (BAK-ter-in): Vaccine made from bacteria.

bacteriology (bak-TEE-ree-**AH**-loh-jee): Study of bacteria.

bacterium, bacteria (pl) (bak-TEE-ree-uhm, bak-TEE-ree-uh): A unicellular microorganism that reproduces by binary fission. They may or may not be pathogenic (cause disease).

bacteriuria (bak-TEE-ree-**YOO**-ree-uh): Bacteria in the urine.

balling gun (BAH-ling guhn): Device for administration of large tablets (boluses) to large animals. Consists of a cylinder at one end, in which the bolus is placed, and a plunger handle at the other end.

bar (bahr): The V-shaped portion of the equine hoof wall that lies on either side of the frog.

barren (BEH-rehn): Unable to bear offspring; sterile.

Key to Pronunciation
a=hat • ah=hot • air=hair • al=bell • ay=day • eh=step • ee-deed • er=hurt
eye=fly • i=bit • oh=boa • too=boot • or=for • ow=cow • oy=joy • th=thin
uh=pup • uu=pull • y=fly • yoo=use • zh=measure

barrier (BEH-ree-er): An obstruction or impermeable membrane or cloth.

barrow (BEH-roh): A castrated male pig.

benign (beh-NYN, bee-NYN): Not malignant; with a favorable prognosis.

bezoar (BEE-zor): Concretion or solid foreign body found in the stomach or intestines.

bi- (by): Prefix meaning 2 or twice.

bicuspid (by-KUHS-pid): Having 2 points or cusps.

bifurcate (by-FER-kayt, BY-fer-kayt): To divide into 2 branches.

bifurcation (BY-fer-KAY-shuhn): Division into 2 branches.

bilateral (by-LA-ter-uul): Occurring on 2 sides.

bile (byl): Fluid, produced in the liver and stored in the gallbladder, that aids digestion by emulsification and absorption of fats.

bile duct (byl duhkt): Duct carrying bile from the liver to the gallbladder and duodenum.

binocular (bi-NAHK-yoo-ler): Pertaining to both eyes; having 2 eyepieces.

biological (BY-oh-LAH-ji-kuul): Medicine prepared from living organisms and their products, including serums, vaccines, antitoxins, bacterins, antigens and toxoids.

biopsy (BY-ahp-see): Removal of a small amount of tissue from the body for examination, usually microscopic.

bitch (bich): A female dog.

bladder (BLA-der): A sac serving as a receptacle for a secretion or excretion. Used alone, it refers to the urinary bladder.

blephar/o (BLEH-fuh-roh): Combining form for the eyelid or eyelash.

blepharitis (BLEH-fuh-RY-tis): Inflammation of the eyelids.

blepharospasm (BLEH-fuh-roh-spazm): The tonic spasm of the muscles of the eyelids, resulting in nearly complete closure of the eyelids.

bloat (bloht): Gaseous distention of the stomach or cecum.

blood (bluhd): Fluid, composed of water, cells, clotting factors and other chemicals, that circulates through arteries, capillaries and veins to supply nutrients and remove waste from tissues.

bloodworms (BLUHD-wermz): Worms of the class Nematoda, genus *Strongylus*. Specifically refers to *Strongylus vulgaris* found in horses.

boar (bor): An intact (uncastrated) male pig.

bolus (BOH-luhs): Mass of food ready to be swallowed or passing through the intestines; a large pill; a large volume of fluid rapidly given intravenously.

borborygmus (BOR-boh-**RIG**-muhs): Rumbling or gurgling noises caused by the propulsion of gas through the intestines.

bougie (BOO-zhee): Cylindric instrument used to dilate a tubular organ.

bougienage (BOO-zhee-**NAHZH**): The act of dilating a tubular organ, using a cylindric instrument designed for that purpose.

bovine (BOH-vyn): Pertaining to cattle; an ox.

brachycephalic (BRAY-kee-seh-**FAL**-ik): Having a short, wide head. Usually used to describe dogs with shortened faces, such as Bulldogs, Boxers, Boston Terriers and Pugs.

brady- (BRAY-dee): Prefix meaning slow.

bradycardia (BRAY-dee-**KAHR**-dee-uh): Abnormally slow heart rate.

bradyphagia (BRAY-dee-**FA**-jee-uh): Abnormally slow eating.

breast (brehst): Mammary gland of a female; the ventral chest area of birds; the cranial pectoral area of horses.

Key to Pronunciation
a=hat • ah=hot • air=hair • al=bell • ay=day • eh=step • ee-deed • er=hurt
eye=fly • i=bit • oh=boa • too=boot • or=for • ow=cow • oy=joy • th=thin
uh=pup • uu=pull • y=fly • yoo=use • zh=measure

breech (breech): Presentation of the tail end or rear feet of the animal in the birth canal during parturition (birth). If one of the legs is presented, it is called an incomplete breech.

brindle (BRIN-duul): Haircoat color pattern characterized by dark streaks or spots intermixed with brown, tan or white hair.

brisket (BRIS-keht): Area in ruminants that lies between the front legs and extends dorsocranially to include the ventral part of the neck.

bronch/o (BRAHN-koh): Combining form for bronchi.

bronchiectasis (BRAHN-kee-**EHK**-tuh-sis): Chronic dilatation (expansion) of the bronchi.

bronchitis (brahn-KY-tis): Inflammation of the bronchi.

bronchopneumonia (BRAHN-koh-noo-**MOH**-nee-uh): Inflammation of the lungs, originating in the terminal bronchioles, which can fill with exudate.

bronchoscope (BRAHN-koh-skohp): Instrument used to view the interior of bronchi.

bronchoscopy (brahn-KAH-skoh-pee): Examination of the bronchi by use of a bronchoscope.

bronchospasm (BRAHN-koh-spazm): Spasmodic constriction of the bronchi.

bronchus, bronchi (pl) (BRAHN-kuhs, BRAHN-ky): A large air passage in the lungs.

buccal (BUH-kuul): Pertaining to or toward the cheek.

buck (buhk): An intact male goat or rabbit.

bulla, bullae (pl) (BUUL-uh, BUUL-ee): Large vesicle or blister.

burdizzo (ber-DEE-zoh): Instrument used to castrate animals by crushing the vessels in the spermatic cord; emasculatome.

bursa, bursae (pl) (BER-suh, BER-see): Sac-like cavity filled with thick lubricating fluid and situated at places where friction develops, such as around tendons.

C

cachexia (kuh-KEHK-see-uh): State of advanced malnutrition or debilitation.

calculus, calculi (pl) (KAL-kyoo-luhs, KAL-kyoo-ly): A stone or concretion formed inside the body, usually composed of mineral salts.

calf (kaf): A young bovine, less than 1 year old.

calve (kav): To give birth to a calf.

cancer (KAN-ser): A malignant tumor.

canine (KAY-nyn): Pertaining to dogs; a dog.

canine tooth (KAY-nyn tooth): Large fang in carnivores located immediately caudal to the incisors and rostral to the premolars.

cannon bone (KA-nuhn bohn): The third metacarpal bone in the front leg of a horse; the large bone distal to the carpus or "knee" in the front leg of a horse.

canth/o (KAN-thoh): Combining form for canthus.

canthus (KAN-thuhs): The angle formed at the junction of the upper and lower eyelids on the medial and lateral sides.

capillary (**KAP**-i-LEH-ree): Minute vessels connecting arterioles to venules, forming a network in almost all of the tissues of the body.

-capnia (KAP-nee-uh): Suffix relating to carbon.

capon (KAY-pahn): A castrated rooster or other male bird.

caprine (KAY-pryn): Pertaining to goats; a goat.

carcinoid (KAR-si-noyd): Carcinoma-like; a yellow circumscribed tumor that occurs in the small intestine, cecum, appendix, stomach or colon.

carcinoma, carcinomas or carcinomata (pl) (KAHR-si-**NOH**-muh, KAHR-si-**NOH**-muhz, KAHR-si-**NOH**-muh-tuh): An invasive malignant tumor arising from epithelial tissues.

Key to Pronunciation

a=hat • ah=hot • air=hair • al=bell • ay=day • eh=step • ee-deed • er=hurt
eye=fly • i=bit • oh=boa • too=boot • or=for • ow=cow • oy=joy • th=thin
uh=pup • uu=pull • y=fly • yoo=use • zh=measure

cardi/o (KAHR-dee-oh): Combining form for heart.

cardia (KARH-dee-uh): The part of the stomach surrounding the junction between the esophagus and the stomach.

cardiac (KAHR-dee-ak): Pertaining to the heart.

cardiodynia (KAHR-dee-oh-**DY**-nee-uh): Pain in the heart.

cardiologist (KAHR-dee-**AH**-loh-jist): A doctor specializing in diseases of the heart.

cardiology (KAHR-dee-**AH**-loh-jee): Study of the heart and blood vessels.

cardiomegaly (KAHR-dee-oh-**MEH**-guh-lee): Enlargement of the heart.

cardiopathy (KAHR-dee-**AH**-puh-thee): Any disease of the heart.

carditis (kahr-DY-tis): Inflammation of the heart.

carnassial tooth (kahr-NAY-see-uul): The fourth upper premolar or the first lower molar in carnivores.

carnivore (KAHR-ni-vor): Animal that eats flesh or meat.

carp/o (KAHR-poh): Combining form for carpus.

carpus (KAHR-puhs): The joint distal to the radius and ulna, and proximal to the metacarpal bones. In people it is called the wrist and in horses it is the "knee" joint of the front leg.

cartilage (KAHR-ti-lij): Specialized fibrous connective tissue found in the embryo, developing bones and joints.

cast (kast): A stiff dressing or bandage used to immobilize a body part; the act of restraining a large animal in recumbency with ropes; a cylindric mass of cells or debris formed in a tubular structure, such as the renal tubules.

castrate (KAS-trayt): To destroy surgically or remove the testes; a male animal whose testes have been removed or destroyed.

catabolic (KA-tuh-**BAH**-lik): Pertaining to or promoting conversion of tissue or complex compounds into simple compounds.

cataract (KA-tuh-rakt): Opacity of the lens of the eye.

cathartic (kuh-THAHR-tik): Causing evacuation of the bowels; agent that causes evacuation of the bowels.

catheter (KA-theh-ter): A tubular instrument used to withdraw fluid from the body, such as a body cavity or the urinary bladder, or to administer fluids, such as into a vein, artery or body cavity.

caudad (KAH-dad): In the direction of the tail or rear end; caudally.

caudal (KAH-duul): Pertaining to the tail end of the body.

cautery (KAH-teh-ree): Application of a cold or hot instrument, electric current or corrosive substance to stop hemorrhage or destroy tissues.

cec/o (SEE-koh): Combining form for cecum.

cecum (SEE-kuhm): The proximal part of the large intestine, forming a dilated pouch to which the ileum and colon are attached.

-cele (seel): Suffix related to a swelling, tumor or cavity.

celiotomy (SEE-lee-**AH**-toh-mee): Incision into the abdominal cavity.

centesis (sehn-TEE-sis): Perforation or tapping a body cavity or organ using a needle, aspirator or trocar. When it is used as a suffix and affixed to a root word, the body part involved is indicated by the root.

centi- (SEHN-ti): Prefix denoting one one-hundredth (1/100) of a unit.

centigrade (SEHN-ti-grayd): Having 100 divisions or gradations; the Celsius temperature scale, where 0 degrees is the freezing point of water and 100 degrees is the boiling point of water (at sea level).

centimeter (**SEHN**-ti-MEE-ter): 1/100 of a meter.

Key to Pronunciation

a=hat • ah=hot • air=hair • al=bell • ay=day • eh=step • ee-deed • er=hurt
eye=fly • i=bit • oh=boa • too=boot • or=for • ow=cow • oy=joy • th=thin
uh=pup • uu=pull • y=fly • yoo=use • zh=measure

centrifuge (SEHN-tri-fyooj): Machine that spins solutions at very high speeds so as to separate the lighter portions from the heavier portions.

cephal/o (SEH-fuh-loh): Combining form for head.

cephalic (seh-FAL-ik): Pertaining to the head or head end of the body.

cerebell/o (SEH-ruh-**BEH**-loh): Combining form for cerebellum.

cerebellum (SEH-ruh-**BEH**-luhm): A part of the brain that lies caudal to the cerebrum and functions in coordination of movement.

cerebr/o (SEH-ree-broh, seh-REE-broh): Combining form for cerebrum.

cerebrum (SEH-ree-bruhm, seh-REE-bruhm): The main portion of the brain that lies in the rostrodorsal part of the skull and functions in thought, memory and movement.

cerumen (seh-ROO-mehn): Earwax.

ceruminolytic (seh-ROO-mi-noh-**LI**-tik): Agent that dissolves earwax.

cervic/o (SER-vi-koh): Combining form for cervix.

cervix, cervices (pl) (SER-viks, SER-vi-seez): The constricted portion or neck of an organ; the caudal part of the uterus that opens into the vagina.

cheil/o (KY-loh): Combining form for lip.

cheiloplasty (**KY**-loh-PLAS-tee): Surgical repair of a lip defect.

chemotherapy (KEE-moh-**THEH**-ruh-pee): Treatment of disease with chemical agents, especially treatment of cancer.

chestnut (CHEHST-nuht): A small area of a horn-like material found on the medial surface of all 4 legs of a horse, just proximal to the carpus on the front legs and distal to the point of the hock in the rear legs.

chiropractor (**KY**-roh-PRAK-ter): Doctor of chiropractic medicine, a system of manipulative treatment of the spinal column believed to restore normal function of the nervous system.

Chlamydia (kluh-MI-dee-uh): A bacterium-like microorganism that is pathogenic to numerous domestic species of animals.

chlor/o (KLOR-oh): Prefix meaning green.

Chlorobacterium (KLOR-oh-bak-TEE-ree-uhm): A genus of bacteria that contain green pigments.

chlorophyll (KLOR-oh-fil): The green-colored matter inside plant cells by which photosynthesis occus.

choke (chohk): Obstruction of the esophagus, caused by a foreign body, bolus of food or a stricture.

chole-, chol/o (KOH-lee, KOH-loh): Combining forms for bile.

cholecyst/o (KOH-lee-SIS-toh): Combining form for gallbladder.

cholecystectomy (KOH-lee-sis-TEK-toh-mee): Excision of the gallbladder.

cholecystolithotripsy (KOH-lee-SIS-toh-LITH-oh-TRIP-see): Crushing of stones (gallstones) in the gallbladder.

choledoch/o (koh-LEH-doh-koh): Combining form for the common bile duct.

choledochocentesis (koh-LEH-doh-koh-sehn-TEE-sis): To withdraw fluid from the common bile duct.

chondr/o (KAHN-droh): Combining form for cartilage.

chrom/o, chromato- (KROH-moh, kroh-MA-toh): Prefix relating to color.

chromatin (KROH-muh-tin): The readily stainable portion of the nucleus comprising the genetic material of a cell.

chromatology (KROH-muh-TAH-loh-jee): Study of colors.

Key to Pronunciation
a=hat • ah=hot • air=hair • al=bell • ay=day • eh=step • ee-deed • er=hurt
eye=fly • i=bit • oh=boa • too=boot • or=for • ow=cow • oy=joy • th=thin
uh=pup • uu=pull • y=fly • yoo=use • zh=measure

chromorrhinorrhea (KROH-moh-RY-noh-**REE**-uh): Discharge of pigmented (colored) secretion from the nose.

chromosome (KROH-moh-zohm): A structure in a cell nucleus that contains genetic information in the form of DNA.

chronic (KRAH-nik): Persisting over a long period.

cicatrix (SI-kuh-triks): A scar.

cilium, cilia (pl) (SI-lee-uhm, SI-lee-uh): A minute hair-like process attached to the free surface of a cell; an eyelash; the eyelid or edge of the eyelid.

circum- (SER-kuhm): Prefix meaning around or surrounding.

circumanal (SER-kuhm-**AY**-nuul): Around or surrounding the anus.

cirrh- (seer): Prefix meaning yellow-orange.

cirrhosis (see-ROH-sis): A chronic interstitial inflammation of an organ, usually accompanied by a yellow-orange discoloration; often applied specifically to the liver.

cloac/o (kloh-AY-koh): Combining form for cloaca.

cloaca (kloh-AY-kuh): The common opening for the colon, urethra and reproductive tract in birds and egg-laying mammals.

clot (klaht): A semi-solid mass, as of organized blood cells.

coagulation (koh-AG-yoo-**LAY**-shuhn): Clot formation; solidification of a solution into a gelatinous mass.

coccus, cocci (KAH-kuhs, KAHK-sy, KAH-ky): A spherical bacterium.

coccyg/o (kahk-**SI**-joh): Combining form for coccyx.

coccyx (KAHK-siks): Group of vertebrae caudal to the sacrum; vertebrae of the tail.

cock (kahk): A male bird.

coffin bone or joint (KAH-fin bohn or joynt): The third and most distal phalanx in the legs of a horse; the main weight-bearing bone inside the hoof. The coffin joint is the joint between the second and third phalanges.

coitus (KOH-i-tuhs): Sexual union; copulation.

col/o (KOH-loh): Combining form for colon.

colic (KAH-lik): Acute abdominal pain; pertaining to the colon.

colitis (koh-LY-tis): Inflammation of the colon.

collateral (koh-LA-ter-uul): Secondary or accessory; a small side branch.

colonoscopy (KOH-lehn-**AHS**-koh-pee): Examination of the colon with a scope.

colostomy (koh-LAHS-toh-mee): Surgical creation of an opening between the colon and the body surface.

colt (kohlt): An intact male horse under 4 years old.

condition (kahn-DI-shuhn): State of health.

conformation (KAHN-for-**MAY**-shuhn): The shape and arrangement of parts.

congenital (kahn-JEH-ni-tuul): Present at birth.

conjunctiv/o (kahn-JUHNK-ti-voh): The combining form for conjunctiva.

conjunctiva (KAHN-juhnk-**TY**-vuh): Membrane that lines the inner eyelids and covers the exposed surface of the eyeball; sclera.

consolidation (kahn-SAH-li-**DAY**-shuhn): Process or condition of becoming solid.

contact (KAHN-takt): The surface of a tooth facing an adjacent or opposing tooth; direct or indirect exposure of a susceptible animal to a communicable disease.

contra- (KAHN-truh): Prefix meaning against, opposed or opposite of.

contrafissure (KAHN-truh-**FI**-sher): Fracture in a part opposite the site of a blow.

Key to Pronunciation
a=hat • ah=hot • air=hair • al=bell • ay=day • eh=step • ee-deed • er=hurt
eye=fly • i=bit • oh=boa • too=boot • or=for • ow=cow • oy=joy • th=thin
uh=pup • uu=pull • y=fly • yoo=use • zh=measure

contraindication (KAHN-truh-IN-di-**KAY**-shuhn): A circumstance, condition or disease that renders a particular treatment inappropriate or undesirable.

contralateral (KAHN-truh-**LA**-teh-ruul): Pertaining to or situated on the opposite side.

convulsion (kahn-VUHL-shuhn): Violent, involuntary contraction of skeletal muscles, originating from a neurological disorder.

copr/o (KAH-proh): Combining form for feces.

coprophagy (kah-PRAH-fuh-jee): Eating of feces.

copulation (KAHP-yoo-**LAY**-shuhn): Sexual union; coitus.

cornea (KOR-nee-uh): The transparent anterior portion of the fibrous outer tunic of the eye.

cortex (KOR-tehks): Outer layer of an organ or structure.

corticosteroid (KOR-ti-koh-**STEH**-royd): Hormone produced by the adrenal cortex.

cortisol (KOR-ti-sahl): Major hormone produced by the adrenal cortex.

cortisone (KOR-ti-sohn): A major hormone produced by the adrenal gland, from which cortisol is deried.

cost/o (KAH-stoh): Combining form for ribs.

costochondral junction (KAH-stoh-**KAHN**-druul JUHNK-shuhn): Junction between the bony and cartilaginous portions of a rib.

crani/o (KRAY-nee-oh): Combining form for the cranium or skull.

cranial (KRAY-nee-uul): Pertaining to the cranium or head end of the body, or denoting a position toward the cranium or head end of the body.

craniotomy (KRAY-nee-**AH**-toh-mee): Incision into the cranium or skull.

cranium (KRAY-nee-uhm): The skeleton of the head; the skull.

creep (kreep): Structure used to limit access of older livestock to feed so that young animals may feed without competition.

croup (kroop): Area on the dorsal surface of a horse, located between the hip area and the head of the tail.

cryo- (KRY-oh): Prefix relating to cold.

cryocautery (KRY-oh-**KAH**-teh-ree): Destruction of tissue by application of extreme cold.

cryosurgery (KRY-oh-**SER**-jeh-ree): Destruction of tissues by application of extreme cold.

cryotherapy (KRY-oh-**THEH**-ruh-pee): Use of cold for therapeutic purposes.

crypt/o (KRIP-toh): Prefix meaning hidden or concealed.

cryptolith (KRIP-toh-lith): Calculus or concretion in a small pit or tube-like depression.

cryptorchid (krip-TOR-kid): Male in which one or both testes have not descended into the scrotum.

cryptorchidism (krip-TOR-kid-izm): Condition in which one or both testes have not descended into the scrotum.

cud (kuhd): Regurgitated bolus of ingesta chewed by ruminants.

culture (KAHL-cher): A growth of microorganisms on living tissue cells or an artificial medium; to perpetuate microorganisms.

cure (kyoor): Successful treatment of a disease, condition or wound; the course, method, system or remedy used to treat a disease, condition or wound.

cut (kuht): An incision or wound; common term for castration.

cutane/o (kyoo-TAY-nee-oh): Combining form for skin.

cyan/o (sy-A-noh): Prefix meaning blue.

cyanosis (SY-uh-**NOH**-sis): Bluish discoloration of the mucous membranes and skin caused by poor tissue oxygenation.

cyanuria (SY-a-**NOO**-ree-uh): Passage of blue urine.

Key to Pronunciation
a=hat • ah=hot • air=hair • al=bell • ay=day • eh=step • ee-deed • er=hurt
eye=fly • i=bit • oh=boa • too=boot • or=for • ow=cow • oy=joy • th=thin
uh=pup • uu=pull • y=fly • yoo=use • zh=measure

cyst/o (SIS-toh): Combining form for bladder, sac or cyst; most commonly refers to the urinary bladder.

cystocele (SIS-toh-seel): Herniation of the bladder through the vaginal wall.

cystodynia (SIS-toh-**DY**-nee-uh): Pain in the urinary bladder.

cystoscopy (sis-TAHS-koh-pee): Visual examination of the urinary bladder through a scope specifically designed to view the bladder.

cytology (sy-TAH-loh-jee): Study of cells.

cytometer (sy-TAH-meh-ter): Device used to count cells.

cytopenia (SY-toh-**PEE**-nee-uh): Deficiency in certain blood cells.

D

dacry/o (DA-kree-oh): Combining form relating to tears or the lacrimal (tear) gland.

dactyl/o (DAK-ti-loh): Combining form relating to digits or toes.

datum, data (pl) (DAY-tuhm, DAY-tuh): Collection of facts or statistics on which a diagnosis is based or an inference made.

de- (dee): Prefix meaning down, from or loss of.

debride (dee-BRYD): Surgical removal of foreign matter and devitalized tissues from a wound.

deci- (DEH-si): Prefix designating one-tenth.

deciliter (DEH-si-lee-ter): 1/10 of a liter; 100 milliliters; abbreviated dl.

decongestant (DEE-kahn-**JEHS**-tehnt): Agent that reduces swelling or congestion of tissue.

defecation (DEH-feh-**KAY**-shuhn): Natural evacuation of fecal material from the rectum.

dehorn (dee-HORN): To surgically or chemically remove the horns.

dehydrate (dee-HY-drayt): Removal of water from the body.

dehydration (DEE-hy-**DRAY**-shuhn): Condition caused by excessive loss of water from the body.

dent/o (DEHN-toh): Combining form for teeth.

derma-, derm/o, dermat/o (DER-muh, DER-moh, der-MA-toh): Combining forms for skin.

dermatologist (DER-muh-**TAH**-loh-jist): Specialist in diseases of the skin.

dermatology (DER-muh-**TAH**-loh-jee): Study of the skin and its disorders.

dermatome (DER-muh-tohm): Instrument used to cut thin skin slices for skin grafting.

dermatophyte (der-MA-toh-fyt): Fungus that grows on the skin.

dermatosis (DER-muh-**TOH**-sis): Any disease of the skin.

descemet/o (DEH-seh-**MEH**-toh): Combining form for Descemet's membrane.

descemetocele (DEH-seh-**MEH**-toh-seel): Herniation of Descemet's membrane through the exterior of the cornea.

Descemet's membrane (DEH-seh-**MAYZ** MEHM-brayn): Fibrous layer lying between the stroma and endothelium of the cornea.

dewclaw (DOO-klah): The first, nonweight-bearing digit. In dogs and cats, they are located medially, just proximal to the other claws. Cattle, sheep, goats and pigs have them on both sides of their legs.

dewlap (DOO-lap): Loose fold of skin hanging from the neck in certain breeds of cattle.

dia- (DY-uh): Prefix meaning through, apart, across or between.

Key to Pronunciation
a=hat • ah=hot • air=hair • al=bell • ay=day • eh=step • ee-deed • er=hurt
eye=fly • i=bit • oh=boa • too=boot • or=for • ow=cow • oy=joy • th=thin
uh=pup • uu=pull • y=fly • yoo=use • zh=measure

diagnosis, diagnoses (pl) (DY-ag-**NOH**-sis, DY-ag-**NOH**-seez): The documented cause of a disease or condition.

diapedisis (DY-uh-peh-**DEE**-sis): Passage of blood cells outward through an intact vessel wall.

diarrhea (DY-uh-**REE**-uh): Abnormal liquidity of the feces and/or increased frequency of defecation.

diastolic (DY-uh-**STAH**-lik): Pertaining to the time when the heart ventricles are dilated with blood and not contracting.

diestrus (dy-EH-struhs): Short quiescent period between metestrus and proestrus in the estrous cycle.

digit (DI-jit): The toe of an animal; finger or toe of a person.

dilatation (dil-uh-TAY-shuhn): Condition of being stretched and made bigger beyond normal dimensions.

dilation (dy-LAY-shuhn): Action of stretching to make bigger.

diplo- (DI-ploh): Prefix meaning double, twin, 2-fold or twice.

diplobacillus, diplobacilli (pl) (DI-ploh-buh-**SIL**-uhs, DI-ploh-buh-**SIL**-eye): Short, rod-shaped bacterium that occurs in pairs.

diplococcus, diplococci (pl) (DIP-loh-**KAH**-kuhs, DIP-loh-**KAH**-ky): Spherical bacterium that occurs in pairs; bacterium of the genus *Diplococcus*.

diplopia (di-PLOH-pee-uh): Double vision; seeing 2 images of a single object.

Diptera (DIP-teh-ruh): Order of 2-winged insects that includes flies, gnats and mosquitos.

dis- (dis): Prefix meaning reversal, separation, duplication or twice.

disease (di-ZEEZ): Illness; deviation from normal physiologic function.

distal (DIS-tuul): Farther from any point of reference or farthest from the central axis of the body or a body part.

diuresis (DY-yoo-**REE**-sis): Increased production of urine.

diuretic (DY-yoo-**REH**-tik): Agent that increases production of urine.

dock (dahk): Surgical removal of all or part of the tail of an animal.

doe (doh): A female goat.

dolichocephalic (DAH-li-KOH-seh-**FA**-lik): Having a long head, such as in Collies and Greyhounds.

dorsal (DOR-suul): Pertaining to the back or topline area of quadrupeds; denoting a position more toward an animal's back than some other reference point or body part.

dorso-, dorsi- (DOR-soh, DOR-see): Combining form denoting a position more toward the back or spine than some other reference point.

dorsum (DOR-suhm): The back or vertebral area of the body.

dose (dohs): A specified amount of medication or other therapeutic agent.

dosimetry (doh-SI-meh-tree): Determination of the amount of radiation emanating from a source.

drench (drehnch): Administration of liquid medication by pouring it into the mouth from a bottle or with a dose syringe; liquid medication given orally by bottle or dose syringe.

-drome (drohm): Suffix meaning a course, conduction or running.

drug (druhg): Any substance used to prevent, diagnose or treat disease.

dry cow (dry cow): Cow not producing milk.

duoden/o (DOO-oh-**DEE**-noh): Combining form for duodenum.

duodenum (DOO-oh-**DEE**-nuhm, doo-AH-deh-nuhm): Proximal part of the small intestines extending from the pylorus to the jejunum.

Key to Pronunciation
a=hat • ah=hot • air=hair • al=bell • ay=day • eh=step • ee-deed • er=hurt
eye=fly • i=bit • oh=boa • too=boot • or=for • ow=cow • oy=joy • th=thin
uh=pup • uu=pull • y=fly • yoo=use • zh=measure

dwarf (dworf): Abnormally small or undersized animal.

-dynia (DY-nee-uh): Suffix meaning pain.

dys- (dis): Prefix meaning difficult, painful or impaired.

dysfunction (dis-FUHNK-shuhn): Impaired or abnormal function.

dysphagia (dis-FA-jee-uh): Difficulty in swallowing.

dysplasia (dis-PLAY-zhee-uh): Abnormal development in size or shape.

dyspnea (DISP-nee-uh): Difficulty in breathing; labored respirations.

dystocia (dis-TOH-shee-uh): Abnormal labor or difficulty in giving birth.

dystrophy (DIS-troh-fee): Disorder occurring as a result of defective or faulty nutrition of tissues.

dysuria (dis-YOO-ree-uh): Difficult or painful urination.

E

ecchymosis (EH-ki-**MOH**-sis): Small area of hemorrhage in the skin or mucous membrane; an ecchymosis is larger than a petechia.

echocardiogram (EH-koh-**KAR**-dee-oh-gram): Image of heart structures produced by ultrasonic waves.

ect/o (EHK-toh): Prefix meaning outside, outer, without or on the outer part.

-ectasis, -ectasia (EHK-tuh-sis, ehk-TAY-zhee-uh): Suffix meaning dilatation, expansion or distention.

ectoderm (EHK-toh-derm): Outermost of the 3 primary germ layers of the embryo, from which develop the nervous system, skin and external sense organs.

-ectomy (EHK-toh-mee): Excision of an organ or part.

ectoparasite (EHK-toh-**PAIR**-uh-syt): Plant or animal that lives on the skin or in external openings of its host.

edema (eh-DEE-muh): Accumulation of excessive fluid in the spaces between cells of tissue.

efficacy (EH-fi-kuh-see): Ability to produce the desired effects; effectiveness.

eisanthema (eye-ZAN-theh-muh): Eruption of a mucous membrane.

elastrator (ee-LA-stray-tor): Instrument used to apply rubber bands to the base of the scrotum of very young calves and lambs, leading to testicular necrosis.

electrocardiogram (ee-LEHK-troh-**KAHR**-dee-oh-gram): Tracing produced by electrical impulses associated with contraction of the heart muscle.

electrocardiograph (ee-LEHK-troh-**KAHR**-dee-oh-graf): Instrument used to record the electrocardiogram.

electrocardiography (ee-LEHK-troh-KAHR-dee-**AH**-gruh-fee): Procedure of making the tracings produced by electrical impulses associated with heart contraction.

electroencephalography (ee-LEHK-troh-ehn-SEH-fuh-**LAH**-gruh-fee): Procedure of recording the electrical currents produced by the brain.

Elizabethan collar (eh-LI-zuh-**BEH**-thehn KAH-ler): Funnel-shaped sheet of cardboard, plastic or x-ray film placed around an animal's neck to prevent self-mutilation.

emaciation (ee-MAY-shee-**AY**-shuhn): State of extreme weight loss; cachexia.

emasculatome (ee-MA-skyoo-luh-tohm): Instrument used to castrate animals by crushing the vessels in the spermatic cord; burdizzo.

emasculator (ee-**MA**-skyoo-LAY-tor): Instrument used to castrate a large animal by simultaneously crushing and cutting the spermatic cord.

embolism (EHM-boh-lizm): Sudden obstruction of a blood vessel by a clot or foreign material brought to the area by the flow of blood.

Key to Pronunciation

a=hat • ah=hot • air=hair • al=bell • ay=day • eh=step • ee=deed • er=hurt
eye=fly • i=bit • oh=boa • too=boot • or=for • ow=cow • oy=joy • th=thin
uh=pup • uu=pull • y=fly • yoo=use • zh=measure

emesis (EHM-eh-sis, eh-MEE-sis): Act of vomiting.

-emia (EE-mee-uh): Suffix relating to blood, blood cells or the bloodstream.

encephal/o (ehn-SEH-fuh-loh): Combining form for the brain.

encephalitis (ehn-SEH-fuh-**LY**-tis): Inflammation of the brain.

end/o (EHN-doh): Prefix meaning inward, inside or within.

endocarditis (EHN-doh-kahr-**DY**-tis): Inflammation of the endocardium (lining of the heart chambers).

endocardium (EHN-doh-**KAR**-dee-uhm): The membrane lining the inner chambers of the heart and the connective tissue bed on which it lies.

endocrine (EHN-doh-krin): Relating to glands that secrete hormones internally into the blood stream (ductless glands), rather than through a duct.

endocrinologist (EHN-doh-kri-**NAH**-loh-jist): Specialist in ductless glands that secrete hormones internally into the bloodstream.

endocrinology (EHN-doh-kri-**NAH**-loh-jee): Study of the ductless glands that secrete hormones directly into the bloodstream.

endogenous (ehn-DAH-jeh-nuhs): Growing or originating from within an organism.

endometrium (EHN-doh-**MEE**-tree-uhm): Lining of the uterus.

endoparasite (EHN-doh-**PAIR**-uh-syt): Plant or animal that lives within its host.

endotracheal tube (EHN-doh-**TRAY**-kee-uul toob): Flexible tube placed into the trachea through the mouth to administer inhalant gases.

enema, enemas or enemata (pl) (EH-neh-muh, EH-neh-muhz, EH-neh-**MAH**-tuh): Liquid injected into the rectum to stimulate bowel movement. Radiopaque contrast medium is injected to make the rectum and colon more visible by radiography.

enter/o (EHN-teh-roh): Combining form for intestines.

enterolithotripsy (EHN-teh-roh-**LITH**-oh-**TRIP**-see): Crushing a stone or concretion in the intestines.

enterostasis (EHN-teh-roh-**STAY**-sis): Cessation or slowing of intestinal contractions; ileus.

enterotomy (EHN-teh-**RAH**-toh-mee): Incision into the intestine.

entrails (EHN-traylz): Internal organs of animals.

enucleation (ee-NOO-klee-**AY**-shuhn): Removal of the eyeball after cutting the muscles and optic nerve; removal of an entire organ or tumor in such a manner that it comes out clean and whole.

enzootic (EHN-zoh-**AH**-tik): Being present in an animal community at all times but causing few cases of illness.

enzyme (EHN-zym): A protein that can greatly accelerate a chemical or physiologic reaction.

epi- (EH-pi): Prefix meaning on or upon.

epidermis (EH-pi-**DER**-mis): The most superficial, nonvascular layer of the skin.

epididym/o (EH-pi-**DI**-di-moh): Combining form for epididymis.

epididymis (EH-pi-**DI**-di-mis): Coiled duct on the caudal border of the testis in which spermatozoa are stored.

epiglott/o (EH-pi-**GLAH**-toh): Combining form for epiglottis.

epiglottis (EH-pi-**GLAH**-tis): Lid-like cartilaginous structure that covers the opening to the larynx during swallowing.

epilepsy (**EH**-pi-LEHP-see): Disturbance of brain function characterized by intermittent periods of seizure activity, loss of consciousness or other neurologic abnormalities.

Key to Pronunciation

a=hat • ah=hot • air=hair • al=bell • ay=day • eh=step • ee-deed • er=hurt
eye=fly • i=bit • oh=boa • too=boot • or=for • ow=cow • oy=joy • th=thin
uh=pup • uu=pull • y=fly • yoo=use • zh=measure

epiphys, epiphysi/o (eh-PI-fis, EH-pi-**FI**-zee-oh): Combining forms for epiphysis.

epiphysis (eh-PI-fi-sis): End of a long bone and margin of a flat bone.

episi/o (eh-PEE-zee-oh): Combining form for the vulva.

epistaxis (EH-pi-**STAK**-sis): Nosebleed; hemorrhage from the nose.

epizootic (EH-pi-zoh-**AH**-tik): Attacking many animals in an area at one time.

equine (EE-kwyn): Pertaining to horses; a horse.

ergot (ER-gaht): Small mass of horn-like material located in the tuft of hair at the flexion surface of the fetlock joint in horses; portion of a mold that grows on certain cereal grains.

eructate (ee-RUHK-tayt): To belch gas from the stomach.

eruption (ee-RUHP-shuhn): Becoming visible or breaking through, such as a new tooth breaking through gum tissues; area of redness on the skin; a rash.

erythr/o (eh-RI-throh): Prefix meaning red.

erythrocyte (eh-RI-throh-syt): Red blood cell.

erythrocytosis (eh-RI-throh-sy-**TOH**-sis): Increased number of red blood cells.

erythroderma (eh-RI-throh-**DER**-muh): Abnormal redness of the skin.

erythrometer (EH-ri-**THRAH**-meh-ter): Color scale or instrument used to measure degree of redness.

Escherichia (EHSH-er-**EE**-kee-uh): Genus of Gram-negative, rod-shaped bacteria.

-esis (EE-sis): Suffix meaning state or condition.

esophag/o (eh-SAH-fuh-goh): Combining form for esophagus.

esophagotomy (eh-SAH-fuh-**GAH**-toh-mee): Incision into the esophagus.

esophagus (eh-SAH-fuh-guhs): Passage extending from the pharynx to the stomach, through which food passes from the mouth to the stomach.

esthesi/o (ehs-THEE-zee-oh): Prefix relating to feeling or the senses.

esthesia (ehs-THEE-zee-uh): Feeling, sensation or perception.

esthesiogenic (ehs-THEE-zee-oh-**GEH**-nik): Producing sensation.

esthesioneurosis (ehs-THEE-zee-oh-noo-**ROH**-sis): Any disorder of sensory nerves.

estrous (EHS-truhs): Pertaining to estrus.

estrus (EHS-truhs): The cyclic period of sexual receptivity in female mammals, characterized by intense sexual urge.

eu- (yoo): Prefix meaning good, easily or well (as in normal).

euphoria (yoo-FOH-ree-uh): Sense of well-being; absence of pain or distress.

eupnea (YOOP-nee-uh): Normal or easy respirations.

eustachian (yoo-STAY-shee-uhn): Tube connecting the nasopharynx to the middle ear.

euthanasia (YOO-thuh-**NAY**-zee-uh): Easy or painless death.

eutocia (yoo-TOH-shee-uh): Normal labor or bith.

eversion (ee-VER-zhuhn): Turning inside out.

eviscerate (ee-VI-seh-rayt): To remove the viscera or intestinal organs.

ex/o (EHK-soh, EHG-zoh): Prefix meaning outside or outward.

exacerbation (ehg-ZA-ser-**BAY**-shuhn): Increase in severity or clinical signs of a disease or condition.

excise (ehk-SYZ): To cut out or off; to remove surgically.

excretion (ehks-KREE-shuhn): Act of removing or discharging products from the body, such as urine or perspiration; material that is excreted or discharged.

Key to Pronunciation
a=hat • ah=hot • air=hair • al=bell • ay=day • eh=step • ee-deed • er=hurt
eye=fly • i=bit • oh=boa • too=boot • or=for • ow=cow • oy=joy • th=thin
uh=pup • uu=pull • y=fly • yoo=use • zh=measure

exhale (EHKS-hayl, ehks-HAYL): To expel from the lungs by breathing.

exocrine (EHG-zoh-krin): Pertaining to glands that secrete substances through ducts.

exogenous (ehg-ZAH-jeh-nuhs): Growing or originating from outside an organism.

exophthalmos (EHG-zahf-**THAL**-mohs): Abnormal protrusion of the eyeball.

exoskeleton (**EHG**-zoh-SKAL-eh-tuhn): Rigid outer shell of crustaceans and insects.

expectorant (ehk-**SPEHK**-toh-rehnt): Agent that promotes ejection of mucus and other fluids from the lungs and trachea.

extension (ehks-TEHN-shuhn): Movement in which a flexed limb is straightened; movement by which 2 component parts are pulled apart so as to lengthen the whole part.

extra- (EHKS-truh): Prefix meaning outside of, beyond or in addition to.

extracellular (EHKS-truh-**SEHL**-yoo-ler): Outside of the cell.

F

fallopian tube (fuh-LOH-pee-uhn toob): Tube connecting the ovary and uterus, through which ova are transported; the oviduct.

false ribs (fahls ribz): Ribs that do not attach directly to the sternum, but instead attach by a common costal cartilage.

farrow (FAIR-oh): Act of giving birth in pigs.

febrile (FEEB-ryl): Characterized by fever.

feces (FEE-seez): Waste products discharged from the intestinal tract.

feline (FEE-lyn): Pertaining to cats; a cat.

femor/o (FEH-mor-oh): Combining form for femur.

femoral (FEH-mor-uul): Pertaining to the femur or thigh.

femur (FEE-mer): Bone extending from the pelvis to the knee; also called the thigh bone.

fetlock joint (FEHT-lok joynt): Metacarpal-phalangeal (front leg) and metatarsal-phalangeal (back leg) joints in the horse.

fibrillation (fi-bri-LAY-shuhn): Quivering, incomplete contraction of a muscle or muscle group.

fibul/o (FIB-yoo-loh): Combining form for fibula.

fibula (FIB-yoo-luh): The thin bone of the rear leg between the stifle (knee) and hock joints, lying lateral to the tibia.

filly (FI-lee): Young female horse up to 4 years old or until the animal is first bred.

fistula, fistulae (pl) (FIS-tyoo-luh, FIS-tyoo-lee): Abnormal tract or passage between 2 internal organs, or leading from an internal organ to the body surface. Fistulas are named for the organs they connect.

flank (flank): Lateral part of the animal's body extending from the ribs to the ileum.

flexion (FLEHK-shuhn): Act of bending or condition of being bent.

float (floht): To file off the sharp edges from a large animal's teeth so as to flatten the occlusal surface; device used to file off the sharp edges of a large animal's teeth.

fly (fly): Two-winged flying insect.

foal (fohl): Process of giving birth in horses; horse less than one year of age.

focus, foci (pl) (FOH-kuhs, FOH-sy): Center of a pathologic process.

footrot (FUUT-raht): Necrosis of the hoof in ruminants, caused by infection; paronychia.

Key to Pronunciation
a=hat • ah=hot • air=hair • al=bell • ay=day • eh=step • ee-deed • er=hurt
eye=fly • i=bit • oh=boa • too=boot • or=for • ow=cow • oy=joy • th=thin
uh=pup • uu=pull • y=fly • yoo=use • zh=measure

foramen, foramina (pl) (foh-RAY-mehn, foh-RAH-mi-nuh): Natural opening or passage, especially through a bone.

forelock (FOR-lahk): Lock of hair lying on the forehead of a horse. It is considered part of the mane.

fornix, fornices (pl) (FOR-niks, FOR-ni-seez): An arch-like structure or vault-like space.

founder (FOWN-der): Inflammation of the sensitive structures of the foot in hooved animals; laminitis.

fracture (FRAK-cher): The breaking of a part, especially a bone.

freshen (FREH-shehn): Act of a cow giving birth to a calf, after which lactation begins.

friable (FRY-uh-buul): Easily torn, crumbled or pulverized.

frog (frahg): A V-shaped band of horny tissue on the under-surface of the equine hoof.

fungus, fungi (pl) (FUHN-guhs, FUHN-jy): Plants without chlorophyll, such as molds, yeasts and ringworm fungus.

furball (FER-bahl): A hairball.

G

gait (gayt); Manner of walking, running or moving.

gallbladder (GAHL-bla-der): Pear-shaped reservoir for bile, located near the right medial lobe of the liver.

gaskin (GAS-kin): Area of the hind leg extending from the stifle (knee) to the hock (tarsus).

gastr/o (GAS-troh): Combining form for stomach.

gastrectasia (GAS-trehk-**TAY**-zee-uh): Dilatation of the stomach; bloat.

gastritis (gas-TRY-tis): Inflammation of the stomach.

gastrocnemius (GAS-trahk-**NEE**-mee-uhs): Muscle caudal to the tibia that extends the tarsal joint and flexes the stifle joint; the "calf" muscle.

gastroduodenostomy (GAS-troh-DOO-oh-deh-**NAH**-stoh-mee): Surgical creation of a passage between the stomach and the duodenum.

gastroenterologist (GAS-troh-EHN-teh-**RAH**-loh-jist): Specialist in disorders of the stomach and intestines.

gastroenterology (GAS-troh-EHN-teh-**RAH**-loh-jee): Study of disorders of the stomach and intestines.

gastroenterostomy (GAS-troh-EHN-teh-**RAH**-stoh-mee): Surgical creation of a passage between the stomach and intestine.

gastrojejunostomy (GAS-troh-JEH-joo-**NAH**-stoh-mee): Surgical creation of a passage between the stomach and the jejunum.

gastropexy (**GAS**-troh-PEHK-see): Surgical fixation of the stomach to the abdominal wall.

gastroscope (GAS-troh-skohp): Instrument for viewing the interior of the stomach.

gastrotomy (gas-TRAH-toh-mee): Incision into the stomach.

gavage (guh-VAHZH): Forced feeding via a tube placed in the stomach through the mouth.

geld (gehld): Act of castrating a male horse.

gelding (GEHL-ding): Castrated male horse.

generic (jeh-NAIR-ik): Pertaining to a genus; referring to a drug name not protected by a trademark.

genesis (JEH-neh-sis): Process of originating, forming or developing.

genital (JEH-ni-tuul): Pertaining to reproduction or the reproductive organs.

genitalia (JEH-ni-**TAY**-lee-uh): The reproductive organs.

Key to Pronunciation
a=hat • ah=hot • air=hair • al=bell • ay=day • eh=step • ee-deed • er=hurt
eye=fly • i=bit • oh=boa • too=boot • or=for • ow=cow • oy=joy • th=thin
uh=pup • uu=pull • y=fly • yoo=use • zh=measure

genus, genera (pl) (JEE-nuhs, JEH-neh-ruh): Category in classification of organisms, traditionally written in italics and often followed by the species name.

gerbil (JER-buul): *Gerbillus iateronia*, a small burrowing rodent.

gestation (jehs-TAY-shuhn): Period of embryonic and fetal development from fertilization until birth; period of pregnancy.

giant (JY-ehnt): Animal, person or organism of huge size.

gilt (gilt): Young female pig that has not yet farrowed (given birth).

gingiv/o (JIN-ji-voh): Combining form for gingiva.

gingiva, gingivae (pl) (JIN-ji-vuh, JIN-ji-vee): Mucous membranes and supporting fibrous connective tissue surrounding the gums.

gloss/o (GLAH-soh): Combining form for tongue.

glottis (GLAH-tis): The opening between the vocal cords.

gnat (nat): Small winged insect that commonly parasitizes livestock.

gnath/o (NA-thoh): Combining form for jaw.

-gnos (nohs): Suffix meaning to know, known or knowledge.

gonad (GOH-nad): The ovary in females or testes in males.

graft (graft): Any tissue or organ transplanted to or implanted at another location on the body or another body.

gram, -gram (gram): 15.432 grains or 1/1000 of a kilogram, abbreviated g or gm; suffix meaning a written record or image.

granulation (GRAN-yoo-**LAY**-shuhn): Formulation of a small, round, red, fleshy mass in wounds; an abnormal, small mass of lymphoid tissue.

graph, -graph (graf): Diagram or curve representing a calculation, experimental data or clinical values; suffix referring to an instrument for writing or recording.

-graphy (GRA-fee): Suffix meaning the act of writing or recording.

grave (grayv): Very serious or severe.

gravid (GRA-vid): Pregnant; containing developing young.

gum (guhm): Common term for the gingiva of the oral cavity.

gyn-, gyne-, gyno-, gyneco- (jyn, jyn, GY-noh, GY-neh-koh): Combining forms meaning female.

gynecologist (GY-neh-**KAH**-loh-jist): Physician specializing in diseases of the genital tract of women.

gynecology (GY-neh-**KAH**-loh-jee): Branch of human medicine involving disease of the genital tract of women.

gyrus, gyri (pl) (JY-ruhs, JY-ry): One of the ridges, or tortuous elevations of the surface of the brain (cerebrum), caused by an infolding of the cortex during development.

H

hairball (HAIR-bahl): Loose clump of hair (or fur), food and other debris in the stomach. May solidify to become a bezoar.

heart (hahrt): Muscular organ in the thoracic cavity that pumps the blood throughout the body.

heat (heet): Common name for estrus.

hecto- (HEHK-toh): Prefix designating 100.

hectogram (HEHK-toh-gram): 100 grams; 1/10 of a kilogram.

heifer (HEH-fer): Young female cow that has not yet given birth to a calf.

hem/o, hema-, hemat/o (HEE-moh, HEE-muh, hee-MA-toh): Combining form for blood.

Key to Pronunciation
a=hat • ah=hot • air=hair • al=bell • ay=day • eh=step • ee-deed • er=hurt
eye=fly • i=bit • oh=boa • too=boot • or=for • ow=cow • oy=joy • th=thin
uh=pup • uu=pull • y=fly • yoo=use • zh=measure

hemacytometer, hemocytometer (HEE-muh-sy-**TAH**-meh-ter, HEE-moh-sy-**TAH**-meh-ter): Electronic instrument or calibrated glass chamber used to count blood cells.

hematinic (HEE-muh-**TI**-nik): Pertaining to hematin or heme; agent that improves the quality of the blood by increasing the hemoglobin content and number of erythrocytes.

hematocrit (hee-MA-toh-krit): Packed cell volume; volume percentage of red blood cells in whole blood.

hematology (HEE-muh-**TAH**-loh-jee): Study of blood and blood-forming tissues.

hematoma (HEE-muh-**TOH**-muh): Localized collection of blood in an organ, space or tissue.

hematuria (HEE-muh-**TOO**-ree-uh): Blood in the urine.

hemi- (HEH-mee): Prefix meaning half or on one side.

hemilaminectomy (HEH-mee-LA-mi-**NEHK**-toh-mee): Removal of the lamina or wall on one side of a vertebra.

hemiparesis (HEH-mee-pair-**EE**-sis): Weakness or partial paralysis on one side of the body.

hemiplegia (HEH-mee-**PLEE**-jee-uh): Paralysis on one side of the body.

hemoglobin (**HEE**-moh-GLOH-bin): The oxygen-carrying pigment of red blood cells.

hemolysis (hee-MAH-li-sis): Liberation of hemoglobin by rupture of red blood cells.

hemorrhage (HEH-mor-ij): Escape of blood from a vessel; bleeding.

hemospermia (HEE-moh-**SPER**-mee-uh): Blood in the semen.

hemostasis (HEE-moh-**STAY**-sis): Arrest of bleeding.

hemostat (HEE-moh-stat): Instrument used to clamp blood vessels to stop bleeding; agent that stops bleeding.

hemostatic (HEE-moh-**STA**-tik): Agent that stops bleeding.

hemothorax (HEE-moh-**THOR**-aks): Accumulation of blood in the pleural cavity.

hepat/o (heh-PA-toh): Combining form for liver.

hepatitis (HEH-puh-**TY**-tis): Inflammation of the liver.

hepatoma (HEH-puh-**TOH**-muh): A tumor of the liver.

hepatomegaly (heh-PA-toh-**MEH**-guh-lee): Enlargement of the liver.

hepatorrhaphy (HEH-puh-**TOR**-uh-fee): Suturing the liver to repair defect.

hepatosis (HEH-puh-**TOH**-sis): Any disorder of the liver.

hernia (HER-nee-uh): Protrusion of an organ or tissue through an abdominal opening.

herniorrhaphy (HER-nee-**OR**-uh-fee): Surgical repair of a hernia.

heter/o (HEH-teh-roh): Prefix meaning other or another.

heterochromia (HEH-teh-roh-**KROH**-mee-uh): Diversity of color in a part or parts that normally are of one color.

heterosexual (HEH-teh-roh-**SEK**-shoo-uul): Pertaining to the opposite sex; preferring the opposite sex.

heterotransplant (HEH-teh-roh-**TRANZ**-plant): Transplant or graft of tissue between different species; a heterograft; a xenograft.

hip dysplasia (hip dis-PLAY-zhee-uh): Malformation of the hip joint, characterized by poor articulation of the femoral head with the acetabulum, leading to arthritis.

hist/o (HIS-toh): Combining form for tissue.

histamine (HIS-tuh-meen): Naturally occurring substance found in all body tissues that causes dilation of capillaries, smooth muscle contraction, increased gastric secretions and

---

Key to Pronunciation

a=hat • ah=hot • air=hair • al=bell • ay=day • eh=step • ee-deed • er=hurt
eye=fly • i=bit • oh=boa • too=boot • or=for • ow=cow • oy=joy • th=thin
uh=pup • uu=pull • y=fly • yoo=use • zh=measure

increased heart rate. It is a component of the inflammatory reaction.

histology (his-TAH-loh-jee): Study of tissues at the microscopic level.

histopathology (HIS-toh-pa-**THAH**-loh-jee): Study of diseased tissues at the microscopic level.

hostotoxin (HIS-toh-tahk-sin): Substance that is poisonous to tissues.

hives (hyvz): Raised, red patches of skin, often accompanied by itchiness; urticaria.

hock (hahk): The tarsus; the joint distal to the stifle (knee) in the rear leg.

homeo- (HOH-mee-oh): Prefix meaning alike, resembling, always the same, similarity, unchanging or constant.

homeostasis (HOH-mee-oh-**STAY**-sis): Stability of the normal physiologic state.

homeotransplant (HOH-mee-oh-**TRANZ**-plant): Transplant or graft of tissue between individuals of the same species; a homograft; an allograft.

homo- (HOH-moh): Prefix meaning the same.

homodont (HOH-moh-dahnt): Having only one type of teeth.

homograft (HOH-moh-graft): Graft or transplant of tissue between individuals of the same species; a homeotransplant; an allograft.

hoofknife (HUUF-nyf): Instrument used to pare away horny tissue from a large animal's hoof.

hormone (HOR-mohn): Substance produced by an organ causing a specific effect on other organs or tissues.

hornfly (HORN-fly): *Hematobia irritans*, a blood-sucking fly that parasitizes livestock.

host (hohst): Animal or plant that harbors another organism (parasite), providing it with nourishment.

humer/o (HYOO-meh-roh): Combining form for humerus.

humerus (HYOO-meh-ruhs): Front leg bone between the scapula and radius.

hybrid (HY-brid): Organism produced from parents of different strains, varieties or species.

hydro- (HY-droh): Prefix relating to water or hydrogen.

hydrocele (HY-droh-seel): Collection of fluid in a cavity, especially in a cavity formed between the membranes of the spermatic cord.

hydrophobia (HY-droh-**FOH**-bee-uh): Fear of water; common name for rabies.

hydroscope (HY-droh-skohp): Instrument to detect water.

hydrotherapy (HY-droh-**THEH**-ruh-pee): Use of water in treatment of disease.

hyper- (HY-per): Prefix meaning excessive, beyond or above.

hyperadrenocorticism (HY-per-a-DREH-noh-**KOR**-ti-sizm): Condition resulting from excessive secretion of hormones from the cortex of the adrenal glands.

hyperalgia (HY-per-**AL**-jee-uh): Extreme sensitivity to pain; hyperalgesia.

hypercapnia (HY-per-**KAP**-nee-uh): Excessive carbon dioxide in the blood.

hyperesthesia (HY-per-ehs-**THEE**-zhee-uh): Increased sensitivity to stimulation.

hyperplasia (HY-per-**PLAY**-zhee-uh): Abnormally increased numbers of normal cells in a normal arrangement in tissues.

hypertension (HY-per-**TEHN**-shuhn): Persistently high arterial blood pressure.

hyperthermia (HY-per-**THER**-mee-uh): Abnormally high body temperature.

Key to Pronunciation

a=hat • ah=hot • air=hair • al=bell • ay=day • eh=step • ee-deed • er=hurt
eye=fly • i=bit • oh=boa • too=boot • or=for • ow=cow • oy=joy • th=thin
uh=pup • uu=pull • y=fly • yoo=use • zh=measure

hypertonic (HY-per-**TAH**-nik): Increased tone or tension; of higher osmotic pressure than a solution to which it is being compared.

hypertrophy (hy-**PER**-troh-fee): Abnormal growth of an organ or tissue through increased size of its constituent cells.

hypo- (HY-poh): Prefix meaning deficient, beneath or under.

hypocapnia (HY-poh-**KAP**-nee-uh): Deficiency of carbon dioxide in the blood.

hypomotility (HY-poh-moh-**TIL**-i-tee): Deficient movement of a part.

hypoplasia (HY-poh-**PLAY**-zhee-uh): Incomplete development of a body part.

hypotension (HY-poh-**TEHN**-shuhn): Abnormally low blood pressure.

hypothermia (HY-poh-**THER**-mee-uh): Abnormally low body temperature.

hypoxia (hy-**PAHK**-see-uh): Reduced oxygen supply to tissues.

hyster/o (HIS-teh-roh): Combining form for uterus.

hysterectomy (HIS-teh-**REHK**-toh-mee): Excision of the uterus.

I

-ia (ee-uh): Suffix indicating state or condition.

-iasis (**EYE**-uh-sis): Suffix meaning a process or condition resulting therefrom.

iatrogenic (EYE-at-roh-**JEH**-nik): Resulting from the actions of treatment.

icterus (**IK**-ter-uhs): Yellow discolorations of the skin and mucous membranes caused by deposition of bile pigments; jaundice.

idiopathic (ID-ee-oh-**PATH**-ik): Of unknown cause.

idiosyncratic (ID-ee-oh-sin-**KRA**-tik): Pertaining to susceptibility to an adverse reaction from a drug or agent in an individual.

ile/o (IL-ee-oh): Combining form for ileum.

ileotomy (IL-ee-**AH**-toh-mee): Incision into the ileum.

ileum (IL-ee-uhm): Distal portion of the small intestine, between the jejunum and the cecum.

ileus (IL-ee-uhs): Obstruction of the intestines from mechanical, neurologic, muscular or other causes; enterostasis.

ili/o (IL-ee-oh): Combining form for ilium.

ilium (IL-ee-uhm): The broad, most cranial bone of the pelvis.

immune (i-MYOON): Highly resistant to disease because of formation of antibodies.

immunoglobulin (IM-yoo-noh-**GLAHB**-yoo-lin): Protein with antibody activity, synthesized by lymphocytes and plasma cells.

in situ (in-SEE-too): In the normal or natural place.

in utero (in YOO-teh-roh): Within the uterus.

in vitro (in VEE-troh): Within a test tube or other artificial environment, outside the living body.

in vivo (in VEE-voh): Inside the living body.

inbreeding (IN-bree-ding): Mating of closely related animals with similar genetic constitutions, such as mother to son or brother to sister.

incise (in-SYZ): To cut.

incision (in-SI-zhuhn): Wound produced by a sharp instrument.

incisor (in-SY-zer): Blade-like front tooth adapted for cutting.

Key to Pronunciation
a=hat • ah=hot • air=hair • al=bell • ay=day • eh=step • ee-deed • er=hurt
eye=fly • i=bit • oh=boa • too=boot • or=for • ow=cow • oy=joy • th=thin
uh=pup • uu=pull • y=fly • yoo=use • zh=measure

incontinent (in-KAHN-ti-nehnt): Unable to control urination or defecation.

incubation (IN-kyoo-**BAY**-shuhn): Development of microorganisms in a host or culture medium; development of the embryo in the eggs of animals.

incubator (**IN**-kyoo-BAY-tor): Environmentally controlled chamber for incubation of cultures, eggs or living cells, or treatment of neonatal or sick animals.

infection (in-FEHK-shuhn): Invasion of the body by microorganisms.

infectious (in-FEHK-shuhs): Caused by or capable of being communicated by infection.

inflammation (IN-fluh-**MAY**-shuhn): Localized tissue response to injury, characterized by heat, swelling, redness, pain and loss of function.

influenza (IN-floo-**EHN**-zuh): Acute viral respiratory infection; "flu."

infra- (IN-fruh): A prefix meaning beneath, below, situated under or occurring beneath.

infratracheal (IN-fruh-**TRAY**-kee-uul): Beneath the trachea.

infusion (in-FYOO-zhuhn): Introduction of fluid, other than blood, by gravity flow into a vein.

inhale (IN-hayl, in-HAYL): To take into the lungs by breathing.

injection (in-JEHK-shuhn): Introduction of a fluid, by force, into a vessel or part.

insufflation (IN-suh-**FLAY**-shuhn): Blowing a powder, vapor or gas into a passage or cavity.

intact (in-TAKT): State of being sexually whole, and not spayed or castrated.

integument (in-TEHG-yoo-mehnt): The skin.

inter- (IN-ter): Prefix meaning between, or situated, formed or occurring between elements indicated by the root word to which this prefix is attached.

intercostal (IN-ter-**KAH**-stuul): Between the ribs.

interdigital (IN-ter-**DI**-ji-tuul): Between the digits.

intern (IN-tern): Graduate of a veterinary or medical school in their first year of training in a teaching hospital.

internal medicine (in-TER-nuul MEH-di-sin): Specialty dealing with disorders of the internal body systems, including such subspecialties as neurology, cardiology and gastro-enterology.

internist (in-TER-nist): Specialist in internal medicine.

intestine (in-TEHS-tin): Portion of the digestive tract extending from the pylorus to the anus; the bowel.

intra- (IN-truh): Prefix meaning within, inside of, or situated, formed or occurring within the object indicated by the root word to which this prefix is attached.

intramuscular (IN-truh-**MUHS**-kyoo-ler): Situated within the substance of a muscle.

intraoperative (IN-truh-**AH**-per-uh-tiv): Occurring during surgery.

intravenous (IN-truh-**VEE**-nuhs): Within a vein.

intubate (IN-too-bayt): To insert a tube into a body canal or hollow organ, such as the trachea or stomach.

intussusception (IN-tuh-suhs-**SEHP**-shuhn): Telescoping of a segment of bowel upon itself.

invertebrate (in-VER-teh-brayt): Any animal with no spinal column.

ipsi- (IP-si): Prefix meaning same.

Key to Pronunciation

a=hat • ah=hot • air=hair • al=bell • ay=day • eh=step • ee-deed • er=hurt
eye=fly • i=bit • oh=boa • too=boot • or=for • ow=cow • oy=joy • th=thin
uh=pup • uu=pull • y=fly • yoo=use • zh=measure

ipsilateral (IP-si-**LA**-teh-ruul): On the same side.

ir-, irid/o (eer, EER-id-oh): Combining forms for iris.

iris (EYE-ris): Colored membrane caudal to the cornea, perforated by the pupil.

irradiation (i-RAY-dee-**AY**-shuhn): Treatment or exposure to ionizing radiation.

irrigate (EER-i-gayt): To wash out or flush; lavage.

ischi/o (IS-kee-oh, I-shee-oh): Combining form for ischium.

ischium (IS-kee-uhm, I-shee-uhm): Most caudal bone of the pelvis.

-ism (izm): Suffix meaning a state or condition.

iso- (EYE-soh): Prefix meaning equal, alike, same as or having the same.

isothermic (EYE-soh-**THER**-mik): Having equal temperatures.

isotonic (EYE-soh-**TAH**-nik): Having equal tone or equal osmotic pressure.

-itis (EYE-tis): Suffix denoting inflammation of the part indicated by the root word to which this prefix is attached.

J

jack (jak): An intact male donkey.

jaundice (JAHN-dis): Yellow discoloration of the skin and mucous membranes caused by deposition of bile pigments; icterus.

jejun/o (jeh-JOO-noh): Combining form for jejunum.

jejunum (jeh-JOO-nuhm): Main part of the small intestines, extending from the duodenum to the ileum.

jennet (JEH-nit): A female donkey.

joint (joynt): Junction between bones; an articulation.

juvenile (JOO-veh-nyl): Pertaining to youth or immaturity.

K

kerat/o (kair-A-toh): Combining form for cornea or horny tissue.

keratitis (KAIR-uh-**TY**-tis): Inflammation of the cornea.

kid (kid): Process of giving birth in goats; a young goat.

kidney (KID-nee): A paired organ, located in the lumbar region, that filters waste products from the blood to produce urine.

kilo- (KI-loh): Prefix indicating 1000.

kilogram (KI-loh-gram): 1000 grams; 10 hectograms; 2.2 pounds.

kyphosis (ky-FOH-sis): Abnormal dorsal or convex curvature of the spine; hunchback.

L

labi/o (LAY-bee-oh): Combining form for labium.

labile (LAY-byl): Chemically unstable.

labium, labia (pl) (LAY-bee-uhm, LAY-bee-uh): A fleshy border or edge between a mucous membrane and the skin, such as the lip. Specifically used to refer to border surrounding the vulva.

laboratory animal medicine (**LAB**-or-uh-TOR-ee AN-i-muul MEH-di-sin): Branch of veterinary medicine involving such laboratory animals as rats, mice, rabbits, gerbils, hamsters, guinea pigs, dogs, cats and subhuman primates.

lacrimal (LAK-ri-muul): Pertaining to tears.

lamb (lam): Process of giving birth in sheep; young sheep.

lamin/o (LAM-i-noh): Combining form for lamina.

Key to Pronunciation

a=hat • ah=hot • air=hair • al=bell • ay=day • eh=step • ee-deed • er=hurt
eye=fly • i=bit • oh=boa • too=boot • or=for • ow=cow • oy=joy • th=thin
uh=pup • uu=pull • y=fly • yoo=use • zh=measure

lamina (LAM-i-nuh): A thin, flat plate or layer.

laminectomy (LAM-i-**NEHK**-toh-mee): Excision of the arch of a vertebra.

laminitis (LAM-i-**NY**-tis): Inflammation of the sensitive structures of the foot in hooved animals; founder.

lance (lans): To cut open with a pointed knife or scalpel.

lapar/o (LAP-uh-roh): Combining form for the loin or flank; more often used in reference to the abdomen or abdominal wall.

laparoscopy (LAP-uh-**RAH**-skoh-pee): Examination of the interior of the abdominal cavity using an instrument designed for that purpose.

laparotomy (LAP-uh-**RAH**-toh-mee): Incision into and through the flank but often meaning through any point of the abdominal wall.

laryng/o (luh-RIN-goh, luh-RIN-joh): Combining form for larynx.

laryngospasm (luh-RIN-goh-spazm): Spasmodic closure of the larynx.

larynx (LAIR-inks): Musculocartilaginous, tubular structure located cranial to the trachea. It serves as the entrance into the trachea, containing the vocal cords.

lateral (LAT-er-ruul): Denoting a position farther from the medial plane of the body or a structure; pertaining to the side of the body or of a structure.

lavage (luh-VAHZH): To irrigate or flush out an organ, such as the stomach.

leiomyoma (LY-oh-my-**OH**-muh): Benign tumor derived from smooth muscle cells.

leptospirosis (lehp-toh-spy-**ROH**-sis): Infection by *Leptospira* bacteria.

lesion (LEE-zhuhn): Any discontinuity of tissue or loss of function.

lethal (LEE-thuul): Deadly or fatal.

leuk/o (LOO-koh): Prefix meaning white or relating to white blood cells.

leukemia (loo-KEE-mee-uh): Malignant disease characterized by proliferation of leukocyte precursors in the bone marrow and increased numbers of white blood cells in the peripheral blood.

leukocyte (LOO-koh-syt): A white blood cell.

leukocytosis (LOO-koh-sy-**TOH**-sis): Increased numbers of circulating white blood cells.

leukomyelitis (LOO-koh-MY-eh-**LY**-tis): Inflammation of the white matter of the spinal cord.

leukopenia (LOO-koh-**PEE**-nee-uh): Decreased numbers of circulating white blood cells.

leukotoxin (LOO-koh-tahk-sin): Toxin destructive to leukocytes.

ligament (LI-guh-mehnt): Band of dense fibrous tissue connecting bones and supporting joints.

ligate (LY-gayt): To tie off.

ligature (LI-guh-cher): Material used to tie off a vessel.

linea alba (LI-nee-uh AL-buh): the tendinous median line of the ventral abdominal wall separating the rectus muscles; the white line.

lingua, lingu/o (LIN-gwuh, LIN-gwoh): Combining forms for tongue. Lingua as a noun means the tongue.

lingual (LIN-gwuul): Pertaining to the tongue; tooth surface toward the tongue.

lipectomy (li-PEHK-toh-mee): Excision of fatty tissue.

Key to Pronunciation
a=hat • ah=hot • air=hair • al=bell • ay=day • eh=step • ee-deed • er=hurt
eye=fly • i=bit • oh=boa • too=boot • or=for • ow=cow • oy=joy • th=thin
uh=pup • uu=pull • y=fly • yoo=use • zh=measure

lip (lip): the upper or lower fleshy margin of the mouth; the margin of a body part.

lip/o (LY-poh, LI-poh): Combining form for fat.

lipoma (ly-POH-muh): Benign tumor composed of fat cells.

liquefaction (LIK-weh-**FAK**-shuhn): Conversion of material into a liquid form.

liter (LEE-ter): Metric unit of volume equal to 1000 milliliters; 100 deciliters, 1000 cubic centimeters of 1.0567 quarts; abbreviated l or L.

lith-, -lith (lith): Prefix or suffix pertaining to a calculus or concretion.

lithiasis (lith-EYE-uh-sis): Condition characterized by the formation of stones, concretions or calculi. This term is often used as a suffix, with the appended prefix denoting the type or location of the calculi.

lithogenesis (LITH-oh-**JEH**-neh-sis): Formation of calculi or concretions.

litholysis (li-THAH-li-sis): Dissolving of a calculus in the urinary bladder.

lithotripsy (**LITH**-oh-TRIP-seee): Crushing of a stone or calculus within a bladder or hollow organ.

litter (LIT-er): Numerous young born at one time of the same mother.

liver (LIV-er): Large dark-red gland, located in the cranial part of the abdominal cavity adjacent to the diaphragm, responsible for numerous critical metabolic functions.

lockjaw (lahk-jah): Common name for tetanus.

loin (loyn): Area on either side of the vertebral column, between the last rib and the pelvis.

lumbar (LUHM-bahr): Part of the back between the thorax and pelvis.

lumbo- (LUHM-boh): Combining form for lumbar.

lumen, lumina (pl) (LOO-mehn, LOO-mi-nuh): Cavity or channel within a tube or tubular organ.

luminal (LOO-mi-nuul): Pertaining to the lumen of a tubular organ.

lung (luhng): Organ of respiration located in the thoracic cavity.

luxation (luhk-SAY-shuhn): Dislocation.

lymph (limf): Transparent, whitish-yellow liquid derived from tissue fluids.

lymph/o (LIM-foh): Combining form for lymph.

lymphaden/o (lim-FA-deh-noh): Combining form for lymph node.

lymphadenopathy (lim-FA-deh-**NAH**-puh-thee): Any disease of the lymph nodes, often characterized by enlargement.

lymphang-, lymphangi/o (LIM-fanj, lim-FAN-jee-oh): Combining forms for lymph vessels.

lymphatic (lim-FA-tik): Pertaining to a lymph vessel; a lymph vessel.

lysis, -lysis (LY-sis): Destruction of cells.

M

macro- (MAK-roh): Prefix meaning large.

mal- (mal): Prefix meaning bad, diseased or impaired.

malacia, -malacia (muh-LAY-shee-uh): Softening or softness of a part or tissue caused by disease.

malignant (muh-LIG-nuhnt): Tending to become progressively worse and result in death. Often used to define potentially fatal tumors.

Key to Pronunciation

a=hat • ah=hot • air=hair • al=bell • ay=day • eh=step • ee-deed • er=hurt
eye=fly • i=bit • oh=boa • too=boot • or=for • ow=cow • oy=joy • th=thin
uh=pup • uu=pull • y=fly • yoo=use • zh=measure

malocclusion (MAL-oh-**KLOO**-zhuhn): Improper alignment or interdigitation of the upper and lower teeth.

malpresentation (MAL-preh-zehn-**TAY**-shuhn): Abnormal presentation of the fetus in the birth canal.

mamm/o (MAM-moh): Combining form for mammary glands.

mammal (MAM-muul): A warm-blooded vertebrate that has hair and suckles its young.

mammary glands (MAM-meh-ree glanz): Cutaneous glandular structures in the female that secrete milk.

mammography (mam-MAH-gruh-fee): Radiography of the mammary glands.

mandible (MAN-di-buul): The lower jaw bone.

mandibul/o (man-DIB-yoo-loh): Combining form for mandible.

mane (mayn): The long hair growing along the dorsal aspect of the neck of horses, from the poll to the withers.

marrow (MAIR-oh): Soft, jelly-like material that fills the cavities of bones. It is a site of blood cell formation.

mast/o (MAS-toh): Combining form for mammary glands.

mastectomy (mas-TEHK-toh-mee): Excision of mammary tissue.

mastitis (mas-TY-tis: Inflammation of the mammary glands.

maxill/o (MAK-si-loh): Combining form for maxilla.

maxilla (mak-SI-luh): Skull bone forming the upper jaw.

mean (meen): Average; numeric value intermediate between 2 extremes, equal to the sum of the value, divided by the number of values.

meconium (meh-KOH-nee-uhm): the dark-green, mucilaginous first feces of the newborn.

medial (MEE-dee-uul): Denoting a position closer to the median plane of the body or part; toward the middle or median plane.

median (MEE-dee-uhn): The midline of the body; a plane running vertically down the midline of the body, dividing it into equal right and left halves; the middle number of value in a sequence.

medicine (MEH-di-sin): Any drug or remedy; the art or science of treating disease by nonsurgical means.

medium, media (pl) (MEE-dee-uhm, MEE-dee-uh): Nutritive substance used in the culture of microorganisms; substance capable of transmitting impulses.

medulla (meh-DOO-luh): Inner portion of an organ or structure.

medullary (**MED**-yoo-LAIR-ee): Pertaining to the marrow or inner portion of an organ or structure.

mega- (MEH-guh): Prefix meaning of great size or enlarged; unit of measure meaning one million times the unit designated by the root with which this prefix is combined.

megacolon (**MEH**-guh-KOH-luhn): An abnormally enlarged or dilated colon.

megaesophagus (MEH-guh-eh-**SAH**-fuh-guhs): Condition in which the esophagus is abnormally enlarged or dilated.

megal/o (MEH-guh-loh): Prefix meaning of great size.

megalocardia (MEH-guh-loh-**KAHR**-dee-uh): Enlargement of the heart; cardiomegaly.

megalohepatia (MEHG-guh-loh-heh-**PA**-tee-uh): Englargement of the liver; hepatomegaly.

-megaly (MEH-guh-lee): Suffix meaning abnormally large or enlargement of the structure indicated by the root word to which this suffix is attached.

Key to Pronunciation
a=hat • ah=hot • air=hair • al=bell • ay=day • eh=step • ee-deed • er=hurt
eye=fly • i=bit • oh=boa • too=boot • or=for • ow=cow • oy=joy • th=thin
uh=pup • uu=pull • y=fly • yoo=use • zh=measure

melan/o (MEH-luh-noh): Prefix meaning black or relating to melanin, a dark body pigment, found in skin, hair, some tumors, the eye, brain and other tissues.

melanocyte (meh-**LA**-noh-syt): Cell that produces melanin.

melanoma (MEH-luh-**NOH**-muh): Tumor comprised of cells containing melanin.

mening/o (meh-NIN-goh, meh-NIN-joh): Combining form for meninges.

meningitis (MEH-nin-**JY**-tis): Inflammation of the membranes enveloping the brain or spinal cord.

meninx, meninges (pl) (MEH-ninks, meh-NIN-jeez): A membrane; the membranes that envelop the spinal cord and brain.

menisc/o (meh-NIS-koh): Combining form for meniscus.

meniscectomy (MEH-ni-**SEHK**-toh-mee): Excision of a meniscus from a joint.

meniscus, menisci (pl) (meh-NIS-kuhs, meh-NIS-ky): Two crescent-shaped fibrocartilaginous pads in the stifle joint; the bulging, crescent-shaped top surface of a liquid in a tube.

mes/o (MEH-zoh): Prefix meaning middle or intermediate, or relating to a mesentery.

mesentery (MEH-zen-teh-ree): Membranous fold of peritoneum attaching the small intestine to the body wall.

mesial (MEE-zee-uul): Toward the median plane of the dental arch.

mesometrium (MEH-zoh-**MEE**-tree-uhm): Part of the broad ligament that suspends the uterus from the dorsal body wall.

meta-, met- (MEH-tuh, meht): Prefix meaning change, transformation after or next.

metabolic (MEH-tuh-**BAH**-lik): Pertaining to the physiologic processes by which cells and tissues are produced and maintained.

metacarpus (MEH-tuh-**KAHR**-puhs): The bones or area immediately distal to the carpus.

metastasis (meh-TAS-tuh-sis): Transfer of disease from one organ or area of the body to another not directly linked to it. Often used to denote spread of tumor cells.

metatarsus (MEH-tuh-**TAHR**-suhs): The bones or area immediately distal to the tarsus.

meter, -meter (MEE-ter, MEH-ter): Basic unit of metric linear measurement equal to approximately 39.37 inches or 1000 millimeters; instrument used in measuring.

metestrus (meht-EHS-truhs): Period after estrus, when the corpus luteum is functional but the female is no longer sexually receptive to males.

metr/o (MEH-troh): Combining form for uterus.

metrorrhagia (MEH-troh-**RA**-jee-uh): Uterine bleeding.

-metry (MEH-tree): Suffix meaning the act of measuring.

micro- (MY-kroh): Prefix designating small size; to indicate one-millionth (10^{-6}) of the unit designated by the root word with which it is combined; abbreviated μ.

microbiologist (MY-kroh-by-**AH**-loh-jist): Specialist in microorganisms.

microbiology (MY-kroh-by-**AH**-loh-jee): Study of microorganisms, such as bacteria, viruses and fungi.

micrometer (my-KRAH-meh-ter, MY-kroh-mee-ter): Instrument used to measure objects viewed through a microscope; one-millionth of a meter; a micron.

micron (MY-kron): one-millionth of a meter; a micrometer; abbreviated μ or μm.

microorganism (MY-kroh-**OR**-gan-izm): Minute living organism, generally microscopic in size, such as viruses, bacteria, fungi and protozoa.

Key to Pronunciation
a=hat • ah=hot • air=hair • al=bell • ay=day • eh=step • ee-deed • er=hurt
eye=fly • i=bit • oh=boa • too=boot • or=for • ow=cow • oy=joy • th=thin
uh=pup • uu=pull • y=fly • yoo=use • zh=measure

microphthalmia (MY-krahp-**THAL**-mee-uh): Abnormal smallness of one or both eyes.

microphthalmos (MY-krahp-**THAL**-mohs): Abnormal smallness of one or both eyes; also spelled microphthalmus.

microscope (MY-kroh-skohp): Instrument used to view minute objects in detail not possible with the naked eye.

microsurgery (**MY**-kroh-SER-jeh-ree): Surgical dissection of minute structures using a microscope.

microtome (MY-kroh-tohm): Instrument used to cut tissues into very thin slices for microscopic study.

micturition (MIK-too-**RI**-shuhn): Passage of urine; urination.

milli- (MIL-li, MIL-lee): Prefix indicating one-thousandth (10^{-3}) of the unit designated by the root word with which it is combined.

milliliter (**MIL**-li-LEE-ter): 1/1,000 of a liter; abbreviated ml.

miosis (my-OH-sis): Contraction of the pupil.

mnemonic (neh-MAH-nik): Pertaining to promoting memory.

molar (MOH-ler): Pertaining to a mass, not a molecule; caudal tooth adapted to grinding.

mon/o (MAH-noh): Prefix meaning one or single

monocular (mah-**NAHK**-yoo-ler): Having one eyepiece or eye.

monogastric (MAH-noh-**GAS**-trik): Having one stomach.

mononuclear (MAH-noh-**NOO**-klee-er): Having one nucleus.

morbid (MOR-bid): Unhealthy; diseased.

morbidity (mor-BI-di-tee): Ratio of sick to healthy animals in a population.

moribund (MOR-i-buhnd): Dying; near death.

morphology (mor-FAH-loh-jee): Study of form and structure of organisms; form and structure of an organism.

mortality (mor-TAL-i-tee): Death rate; ratio of total deaths in a given population (may or may not be limited to a particular disease) to the total number of animals in a given population.

motor (MOH-ter): Producing movement.

mucilaginous (MYOO-si-**LA**-ji-nuhs): Sticky and slimy.

mucoid (MYOO-coyd): Resembling mucus.

mucopurulent (MYOO-koh-**PYOO**-roo-lehnt): Containing mu- cus and pus.

mucosa (myoo-KOH-suh): Membrane lining tubular organ, such as the alimentary tract; a mucous membrane.

mucous (MYOO-kuhs): Pertaining to or resembling mucus; secreting mucus.

mucus (MYOO-kuhs): The slimy secretion found on mucous membranes.

multi- (MUHL-ti, MUHL-ty): Prefix meaning many or much.

multicellular (MUHL-ty-**SEHL**-yoo-ler): Having many cells.

multifocal (MUHL-ty-**FOH**-kuul): Having more than one focus or center; arising from or pertaining to many foci or centers.

murine (MYOO-reen): Pertaining to rats or mice.

muscle (MUH-suul): Tissue with the ability to contract.

muscul/o (MUH-skyoo-loh): Combining form for muscles.

muscular (MUH-skyoo-ler): Pertaining to muscle; having well-developed muscles.

muzzle (MUH-zuul): The nose and the rostral portions of the upper and lower mouth; device placed around the snout and lower jaw to prevent biting.

my/o (MY-oh): Combining form for muscle.

Key to Pronunciation

a=hat • ah=hot • air=hair • al=bell • ay=day • eh=step • ee-deed • er=hurt
eye=fly • i=bit • oh=boa • too=boot • or=for • ow=cow • oy=joy • th=thin
uh=pup • uu=pull • y=fly • yoo=use • zh=measure

mycology (my-KAH-loh-jee): Study of fungi.

mydriasis (mi-DRY-uh-sis): Extreme dilatation of the pupil.

myel/o (MY-eh-loh): Combining form for bone marrow or the spinal cord.

myelogram (MY-eh-loh-gram): Radiograph of the spinal canal after injection of radiopaque dye; graphic representation of a differential cell count of the cells found on a stained bone marrow smear.

myelography (MY-eh-**LAH**-gruh-fee): Radiography of the spinal canal after injection of radiopaque.

myeloma (MY-eh-**LOH**-muh): Malignant tumor composed of cells normally found in the bone marrow.

myelomalacia (MY-eh-loh-muh-**LAY**-shee-uh): Softening of the spinal cord.

myocardium (MY-oh-**KAHR**-dee-uhm): The muscular layer of the heart wall.

myoma (my-OH-muh): Tumor derived from muscle cells.

myometrium (MY-oh-**MEE**-tree-uhm): The smooth muscle layer of the uterus.

myositis (MY-oh-**SY**-tis): Inflammation of voluntary skeletal muscle.

myring/o (mi-RIN-goh): Combining form for the eardrum or tympanic membrane.

myringoplasty (mi-**RIN**-goh-PLA-stee): Surgical repair of a perforated eardrum.

myringotomy (MI-rin-**GAH**-toh-mee): Incision of the eardrum.

N

nanny (NA-nee): An adult female goat.

nano- (NA-noh): Prefix indicating one-billionth (10^{-9}) of the unit designated by the root word with which it is combined.

nanogram (NA-noh-gram): One-billionth (1/1,000,000,000) of a gram; abbreviated ng.

nape (nayp): The dorsum of the neck.

narc/o (NAHR-koh): Combining form meaning stupor or stuporous.

narcotic (nahr-KAH-tik): Pertaining to or producing stupor or insensibility (narcosis); agent that produces stupor; an opioid.

naris, nares (NEH-ris, NEH-rees): Moist rostral opening of the nasal cavity; the nostril.

natal, -natal (NAY-tuul): Pertaining to birth.

navicular (nuh-VI-kyoo-ler): Pertaining to the navicular bone, the distal sesamoid bone in the horse, which lies caudal to the coffin bone.

nebulization (NEHB-yoo-li-**ZAY**-shuhn): Changing a liquid into a fine mist or spray; treatment with a fine mist.

necr/o (NEH-kroh): Prefix relating to death or dead tissue.

necropsy (NEE-krahp-see): Examination of a body after death. *Necropsy* is the preferred term for examination of animal cadavers, while *autopsy* is the preferred term for examination of human cadavers.

necrosis (neh-KROH-sis): Death of tissue and its component cells.

necrotic (neh-KRAH-tik): Pertaining to or characterized by dead tissue.

necrotoxin (NEH-kroh-TAHK-sin): Substance, produced by certain *Staphylococcus* bacteria, that kills tissue cells.

neo- (NEE-oh): Prefix meaning new or strange.

neogenesis (NEE-oh-**GEH**-neh-sis): Regeneration of tissues.

Key to Pronunciation

a=hat • ah=hot • air=hair • al=bell • ay=day • eh=step • ee-deed • er=hurt
eye=fly • i=bit • oh=boa • too=boot • or=for • ow=cow • oy=joy • th=thin
uh=pup • uu=pull • y=fly • yoo=use • zh=measure

neonatal (NEE-oh-**NAY**-tuul): Pertaining to the first few weeks after birth.

neoplasm (NEE-oh-plazm): Any new or abnormal growth, especially that which is progressive and uncontrolled; a tumor.

nephr/o (NEH-froh): Combining form for kidney.

nephrectomy (neh-FREHK-toh-mee): Excision of a kidney.

nephrolith (NEH-froh-lith): A calculus in a kidney.

nephron (NEH-frahn): The basic anatomic and functional unit of the kidney.

nephropathy (neh-FRAH-puh-thee): Disease of the kidneys.

nephrosis (neh-FROH-sis): Any disease of the kidney, especially a degenerative condition of the renal tubules.

nephrotoxin (**NEH**-froh-**TAHK**-sin): Substance with harmful effects on kidney cells.

nerve (nerv): Cord-like structure, made up of numerous fibers, that carries impulses between the central nervous system and some other part of the body.

neur/o (NOO-roh): Combining form for nerve or the nervous system.

neurectomy (noo-REHK-toh-mee): Excision of part of a nerve.

neurologist (noo-RAH-loh-jist): Specialist in disorders of the nervous system.

neurology (noo-RAH-loh-jee): Study of the brain, spinal cord, and nerves.

neuropathy (noo-RAH-puh-thee): Any functional disturbance of the peripheral nervous system.

neurotripsy (NOO-roh-trip-see): Crushing of a nerve.

neuter (NOO-ter): To castrate or spay an animal; an animal whose gonads have been removed.

noct- (nahkt): Prefix meaning night or darkness.

nocturia (nahk-TYOO-ree-uh): Urinating excessively during the night; nycturia.

nomenclature (**NOH**-mehn-KLAY-cher): A system of names used in describing anatomic structures, organisms and other items.

nucleus (NOO-klee-uhs): Spherical body within a cell containing genetic information.

nullipara (nuh-LI-puh-ruh): Animal or person who has never borne a viable offspring.

nyct/o (NIK-toh): Prefix meaning night or darkness.

nyctophobia (NIK-toh-**FOH**-bee-uh): Excesive fear of darkness.

nycturia (nik-TYOO-ree-uh): Urinating excessivly during the night; nocturia.

O

oblique (oh-BLEEK): At an angle, slanting, inclined or between horizontal and vertical.

obstetrician (AHB-steh-**TRI**-shuhn): Specialist in human pregnancy and care of human infants.

obstetrics (ahb-STEH-triks): Branch of human medicine involving prenatal and postnatal care, and delivery of human infants.

occipital (ahk-SIP-i-tuul): Pertaining to the area of the occiput, located at the back of the head.

occlusal (oh-KLOO-suul): the biting or chewing surface of teeth; toward the plane between the mandibular and maxillary teeth.

occlusion (oh-KLOO-zhun): The act of closing off; an obstruction.

Key to Pronunciation

a=hat • ah=hot • air=hair • al=bell • ay=day • eh=step • ee-deed • er=hurt
eye=fly • i=bit • oh=boa • too=boot • or=for • ow=cow • oy=joy • th=thin
uh=pup • uu=pull • y=fly • yoo=use • zh=measure

ocul/o (AHK-yoo-loh): Combining form for eye.

odont/o (oh-DAHN-toh): Combining form for teeth.

odontalgia (OH-dahn-**TAL**-jee-uh): Pain in a tooth; tooth-ache.

-oid (oyd): Suffix meaning alike, resembling or similar to in form.

olig/o (AH-li-goh): Combining form meaning few or scanty.

-oma (OH-muh): Suffix denoting a tumor or neoplasm.

omas/o (oh-MAY-soh): Combining form for omasum.

omasopexy (oh-**MAY**-soh-PEHK-see): Surgical fixation of the omasum to the abdominal wall or some other tissue.

omasum (oh-MAY-suhm): The third division of the stomach of ruminants, lying between the reticulum and the abomasum.

omentum (oh-MEHN-tuhm): Peritoneal fold between the stomach and nearby organs.

oncologist (ahn-KAH-loh-jist): Specialist in tumors.

oncology (ahn-KAH-loh-jee): Study of tumors.

oncornavirus (ahn-**KOR**-nuh-VI-ruhs): An RNA-containing virus that causes cancer.

onych/o (AH-ni-koh): Combining form for nail, claw or hoof.

onychectomy (AH-ni-**KEHK**-toh-mee): Excision of a claw; declawing.

oophor/o (oh-**AH**-for-oh): Combining form for ovaries.

operation (AH-per-**AY**-shuhn): Surgical procedure.

operative (AH-per-uh-tiv): Pertaining to a surgical pro-cedure.

ophthalm/o (ahf-THAL-moh): Combining form for eye.

ophthalmic (ahf-THAL-mik): Pertaining to the eye; medica-tion used in the eye.

ophthalmologist (AHF-thal-**MAH**-loh-jist): Specialist in dis-eases of the eye.

ophthalmology (AHF-thal-**MAH**-loh-jee): Study of disorders of the eye.

ophthalmoscope (ahf-THAL-moh-skohp): Instrument used to view the interior of the eye.

-opia (OH-pee-uh): Suffix relating to vision.

opioid (OH-pee-oyd): Synthetic drug with narcotic effects but not derived from opium.

or/o (OR-oh): Combining form for mouth.

orchi/o, orchid/o (OR-kee-oh, OR-ki-doh): Combining forms for testes.

orchiectomy (OR-kee-**EHK**-toh-mee): Surgical removal of one or both testes; castration.

orifice (OR-i-fis): The opening, entrance or outlet of a body cavity.

orthopedic (OR-thoh-**PEE**-dik): Pertaining to the skeletal system.

-osis (OH-sis): Suffix meaning a disease or pathologic process.

oste/o (AH-stee-oh): Combining form for bone.

osteolysis (AH-stee-**AH**-li-sis): Dissolution of bone, generally by loss of calcium.

osteomalacia (AH-stee-oh-muh-**LAY**-shee-uh): Softening of bones.

osteomyelitis (AH-stee-oh-MY-eh-**LY**-tis): Inflammation of the bone and marrow, caused by a pyogenic organism.

osteotome (AH-stee-oh-tohm): Instrument used to cut bone.

osteotomy (AH-stee-**AH**-toh-mee): Surgical cutting of bone.

ot/o (OH-toh): Combining form for ear.

Key to Pronunciation

a=hat • ah=hot • air=hair • al=bell • ay=day • eh=step • ee-deed • er=hurt
eye=fly • i=bit • oh=boa • too=boot • or=for • ow=cow • oy=joy • th=thin
uh=pup • uu=pull • y=fly • yoo=use • zh=measure

otic (OH-tik): Pertaining to the ear; medication used in the ear.

otorhinolaryngology (OH-toh-RY-noh-LEH-rin-**GAH**-loh-jee): Study of disorders of the ear, nose and throat.

otoscope (OH-toh-skohp): Instrument used to view the external ear canal and typmanic membrane.

ovari/o (oh-VEH-ree-oh): Combining form for ovaries.

ovariectomy (oh-VEH-ree-**EHK**-toh-mee): Surgical removal of one or both ovaries.

ovariohysterectomy (oh-VEH-ree-oh-HIS-ter-**EHK**-toh-mee): Surgical removal of the ovaries and uterus; spay.

ovary (OH-veh-ree): The gonad or sexual gland of the female, in which ova are formed.

oviduct (OH-vi-duhkt): Tubular passage that carries ova to the uterus.

ovine (OH-vyn): Pertaining to sheep; a sheep.

oviparous (oh-VI-puh-ruhs): Producing eggs from which young are hatched outside the mother's body, as in birds.

ovoviviparous (OH-voh-vy-**VI**-puh-ruhs): Bearing live young that hatch from eggs within the mother's body, as in lizards.

ovum, ova (pl) (OH-vuhm, OH-vuh): The female reproductive cell, an egg.

-oxia (AHK-see-uh): Suffix relating to oxygen.

P

pachy- (PA-kee): Combining form meaning thick.

palat/o (PAL-uh-toh): Combining form for palate. This prefix is sometimes used in place of lingu/o when referring to the lingual surface of maxillary teeth.

palate (PAL-uht): Partition separating the oral and nasal cavities.

palmar (PAHL-mahr): Pertaining to the bottom or undersurface of the front feet of a quadruped.

palpation (pal-PAY-shuhn): Using the hands to feel body parts during physical examination.

palpebra, palpebrae (pal-PEE-bruh, pal-PEE-bree): Eyelid.

pan- (pan): Prefix meaning all.

pancreas (PAN-kree-uhs): Gland, located between the spleen and the duodenum, that produces digestive enzymes, insulin and glucagon.

pancreat/o (pan-kree-A-toh): Combining form for pancreas.

pancreatectomy (PAN-kree-uh-**TEHK**-toh-mee): Surgical removal of the pancreas.

panleukopenia (PAN-loo-koh-**PEE**-nee-uh): Viral disease of cats characterized by decreased numbers of white blood cells; decrease in all of the white blood cell elements of the blood.

panosteitis (PAN-ah-stee-**EYE**-tis): Inflammation of an entire bone.

papilloma (PAP-i-**LOH**-muh): Benign epithelial tumor; wart.

para- (PAIR-uh): Prefix meaning beside, beyond or apart from.

paracentesis (PAIR-uh-sehn-**TEE**-sis): Puncture of a cavity for withdrawal of fluid.

paralysis (pair-AL-i-sis): Loss or impairment of the ability to move body parts.

paramedian (PAIR-uh-**MEE**-dee-uhn): Near the midline or median plane of the body.

parameter (pair-A-meh-ter): A measure or value of a body function.

Key to Pronunciation
a=hat • ah=hot • air=hair • al=bell • ay=day • eh=step • ee-deed • er=hurt
eye=fly • i=bit • oh=boa • too=boot • or=for • ow=cow • oy=joy • th=thin
uh=pup • uu=pull • y=fly • yoo=use • zh=measure

paraparesis (PAIR-uh-puh-**REE**-sis): Weakness or partial paralysis of both rear legs.

paraplegia (PAIR-uh-**PLEE**-jee-uh): Paralysis of both rear legs.

parasite (PAIR-uh-syt): Plant or animal that lives on or in another organism at the expense of the host.

parasiticide (PAIR-uh-**SI**-ti-syd): Agent that is destructive or lethal to parasites.

parasitology (PAIR-uh-si-**TAH**-loh-jee): Study of parasites.

parathyr/o (PAIR-uh-**THY**-roh): Combining form for parathyroid gland.

parathyroid glands (PAIR-uh-**THY**-royd glanz): Four small glands, located near or within the thyroid gland, concerned with calcium and phosphorus metabolism.

parathyroidectomy (PAIR-uh-THY-royd-**EHK**-toh-mee): Excision of the parathyroid gland.

paravertebral (PAIR-uh-ver-**TEE**-bruhl): Beside the vertebral column.

parenteral (pair-EHN-teh-ruul): By a route of administration, such as intravenous, intramuscular, intraperitoneal, subcutaneous, intradermal or intracardiac injection, other than through the alimentary canal.

paresis, -paresis (puh-REE-sis): Slight or incomplete paralysis.

paronychia (PAIR-oh-**NEE**-kee-uh): Inflammation or infection of the claw or hoof; footrot.

-parous (PAIR-uhs): Suffix relating to production of live offspring.

paroxysm (pair-AHK-sizm): Sudden recurrence or intensification of signs; a spasm or seizure.

parturition (PAHR-tyoo-**RI**-shuhn): The act of giving birth.

pastern (PAS-tern): Common name for the area of the first and second phalanges in all 4 legs of horses, between the fetlock and the hoof.

path/o (PA-thoh): Prefix relating to disease.

pathogen (PA-thoh-jehn): A disease-producing microorganism.

pathogenic (PA-thoh-**JEH**-nik): Causing disease.

pathognomonic (PA-thahg-noh-**MAH**-nik): Distinctive or specific to a particular disease, such that a diagnosis may be based on it.

pathologic (PA-thoh-**LAH**-jik): Indicating disease.

pathologist (pa-THAH-loh-jist): Specialist in the changes of structure and function caused by disease.

pathology (pa-THAH-loh-jee): Study of the essential nature of disease, especially the effects of disease on tissue structure and function.

-pathy (PA-thee): Suffix meaning a disease.

pediatrics (PEE-dee-**A**-triks): Branch of veterinary and human medicine dealing with disorders of young animals or children.

pediculosis (peh-DI-kyoo-**LOH**-sis): Infestation with lice.

ped/o, pod/o (PEH-doh, POH-doh): Combining forms for foot.

pelv/o, pelvi/o (PAL-voh, PAL-vee-oh): Combining forms for pelvis.

pelvimetry (pal-VI-meh-tree): Measuring the dimensions and capacity of the pelvis.

pelvis (PAL-vis): The paired hip bones, consisting of the ilium, ischium, pubis and acetabular bones.

Key to Pronunciation
a=hat • ah=hot • air=hair • al=bell • ay=day • eh=step • ee-deed • er=hurt
eye=fly • i=bit • oh=boa • too=boot • or=for • ow=cow • oy=joy • th=thin
uh=pup • uu=pull • y=fly • yoo=use • zh=measure

-penia (PEE-nee-uh): Suffix meaning a deficiency; subnormal numbers.

peracute (PAIR-uh-**KYOOT**): Of extremely rapid onset.

percussion (per-KUH-shuhn): The act of striking the body with light, sharp blows as an aid in assessing underlying parts by the sound obtained.

peri- (PAIR-ee): Prefix meaning around or near.

perianal (PAIR-ee-**AY**-nuul): Located around the anus.

pericardial (PAIR-i-**KAHR**-dee-uul): Pertaining to the pericardium.

pericarditis (PAIR-i-kahr-**DY**-tis): Inflammation of the pericardium.

perinatal (PAIR-i-**NAY**-tuul): Pertaining to the period shortly before and after birth.

perineum (pair-i-NEE-uhm): Area between the anus and scrotum or vulva.

periodontal (PAIR-ee-oh-**DAHN**-tuul): Pertaining to the area around a tooth.

periosteum (PAIR-ee-**AH**-stee-uhm): Fibrous connective tissue covering a bone.

peripheral (peh-RI-feh-ruul): Situated away from the central area of the body or a structure.

peristalsis (PAIR-i-**STAHL**-sis): Contraction by the smooth muscles of the alimentary tract or other tubular organ to propel its contents.

peritone/o (PAIR-i-toh-**NEE**-oh): Combining form for peritoneum.

peritoneal (PAIR-i-toh-**NEE**-uul): Pertaining to the peritoneum.

peritoneal cavity (PAIR-i-toh-**NEE**-uul KAV-i-tee): Space within the abdominal cavity between the viscera and the abdominal wall.

peritoneum (PAIR-i-toh-**NEE**-uhm): Serous membrane that lines the wall of the abdominal cavity and envelops the abdominal organs.

perivascular (PAIR-i-**VAS**-kyoo-ler): Situated around a vessel.

permeable (PER-mee-uh-buul): Permitting passage of a substance; not impervious.

petechia, petechiae (pl) (peh-TEE-kee-uh, peh-TEE-kee-ee): Pinpoint, round hemorrhages on the skin or on a serosal surface. Petechiae are smaller than ecchymoses.

Petri dish (PEH-tree dish): Shallow glass or plastic dish for growing cultures of microorganisms.

-pexy (PEHK-see): Suffix meaning to surgically stabilize an organ or tissue in a certain location.

phag/o (FAY-goh, FA-goh): Prefix relating to eating, ingestion or engulfment.

-phagia, -phagy (FA-jee): Suffix referring to eating or swallowing.

phagocyte (FA-goh-syt): Any cell with the ability to ingest microorganisms, foreign particles or other cells.

phagology (fa-GAH-loh-jee): Study of eating or feeding.

phagophobia (FA-goh-**FOH**-bee-uh): Morbid fear of eating.

phalanx, phalanges (pl) (FA-lanx, fa-LAN-jeez): Toe; distal 3 bones of the foot.

pharmaceutical (FAHR-muh-**SOO**-ti-kuul): Pertaining to drugs; a drug.

pharmacodynamics (FAHR-muh-koh-dy-**NA**-miks): Study of or pertaining to effects of drugs; the mechanism of their action, and their metabolism.

Key to Pronunciation
a=hat • ah=hot • air=hair • al=bell • ay=day • eh=step • ee-deed • er=hurt
eye=fly • i=bit • oh=boa • too=boot • or=for • ow=cow • oy=joy • th=thin
uh=pup • uu=pull • y=fly • yoo=use • zh=measure

pharmacognosy (FAHR-muh-**KAHG**-noh-see): Branch of pharmacology dealing with the features of natural drugs.

pharmacology (FAHR-muh-**KAH**-loh-jee): Study of drugs and their actions.

pharmacy (FAHR-muh-see): Science of preparing and dispensing drugs; shop where drugs are prepared and dispensed; area within a hospital where drugs are prepared and dispensed.

pharyng/o (fuh-RIN-goh, fuh-RIN-joh): Combining form for pharynx.

pharynx (FAIR-inks): Passage between the nostrils and the esophagus and larynx. The portion dorsal to the soft palate is called the nasopharynx, while the oropharynx lies ventral to the soft palate.

phleb/o (FLEH-boh): Combining form for vein.

phlebitis (fleh-BY-tis): Inflammation of a vein.

phobia (FOH-bee-uh): Any excessive or unreasonable fear.

phon/o, -phonia (FOH-noh, FOH-nee-uh): Suffix relating to sound or speech.

phonation (foh-NAY-shuhn): The utterance of vocal sounds.

phonocatheter (FOH-noh-**KA**-theh-ter): Catheter with a microphone at its tip.

phonology (foh-NAH-loh-jee): Study of vocal sounds.

phonophobia (FOH-noh-**FOH**-bee-uh): Morbid fear of sounds or of speaking aloud.

phot/o (FOH-toh): Combining form relating to light.

phyt/o (FY-toh): Combining form relating to plants or vegetable matter.

phytobezoar (FY-toh-**BEE**-zor): Concretion or solid mass of vegetable matter found in the stomach or intestine.

pica (PY-kuh): Craving for unnatural items of food, ravenous eating of nonfood times.

pil/o (PY-loh): Combining form for hair.

pinna (PI-nuh): The flap or projecting portion of the ear.

placenta (pluh-SEHN-tuh): The membranes surrounding the developing fetus in mammals, providing nutrition.

plane (playn): Flat surface determined by 3 points in space; specific level of anesthetic depth defined by the response of the patient.

plantar (PLAN-ter): Pertaining to the bottom or undersurface of the rear feet in quadrupeds.

-plasia (PLAY-zhee-uh): Suffix referring to development relative to numbers of cells.

-plasty (PLA-stee): Suffix meaning surgical shaping.

-plegia (PLEE-jee-uh): Suffix meaning paralysis.

pleur/o (PLOO-roh): Combining form relating to the pleura.

pleura (PLOO-ruh): Serous membrane that lines the thoracic cavity and envelops the thoracic organs.

pleural cavity (PLOO-ruul KAV-i-tee): Space within the thoracic cavity between the thoracic organs and the body wall.

plexus (PLEHK-suhs): Network of nerves, veins or lymphatics.

-pnea (NEE-uh): Suffix relating to breathing.

pneum/o (NOO-moh): Combining form relating to the lungs, or breath.

pneumonia (noo-MOH-nee-uh): Infection of the lungs, with varing degrees of consolidation.

pneumonitis (NOO-moh-**NY**-tis): Inflammation of the lungs.

pod/o (POH-doh): Combining form for foot.

Key to Pronunciation
a=hat • ah=hot • air=hair • al=bell • ay=day • eh=step • ee-deed • er=hurt
eye=fly • i=bit • oh=boa • too=boot • or=for • ow=cow • oy=joy • th=thin
uh=pup • uu=pull • y=fly • yoo=use • zh=measure

polio (POH-lee-oh): Combining form relating to the gray matter of the nervous system.

poll (pohl): The most dorsal point on an animal's head.

poly- (PAH-lee): Prefix meaning many, much or multiple.

polyarthritis (PAH-lee-ahr-**THRY**-tis): Inflammation of more than one joint.

polycythemia (PAH-lee-sy-**THEE**-mee-uh): Increased numbers of red blood cells.

polydactyly (PAH-lee-**DAK**-ti-lee): Presence of extra toes.

polyphagia (PAH-lee-**FA**-jee-uh): Excessive or voracious eating.

polysinusitis (PAH-lee-SY-nuh-**SY**-tuhs): Inflammation of multiple sinuses.

polyunsaturated (PAH-lee-uhn-**SA**-choo-ray-tehd): Characteristic of fatty acid with multiple double and triple bonds between carbon atoms.

polyuria (PAH-lee-**YOO**-ree-uh): Producing large quantities of urine.

porcine (POR-syn): Pertaining to pigs; a pig.

posology (poh-SAH-loh-jee): Study of drug dosages.

post- (pohst): Prefix meaning after or behind.

post mortem (pohst MOR-tehm): After death. When used as an adverb, it is correctly written as post mortem. When used as an adjective, it is written postmortem.

posterior (pah-STEE-ree-or): Pertaining to the caudal, rear or back part of the body or a part. In veterinary medicine it is primarily used in descriptions of the eye.

postnasal (pohst-NAY-suul): Situated or occurring caudal to the nose or nasal passages.

postoperative (pohst-AH-per-uh-tiv): Occurring after surgery.

postprandial (pohst-PRAN-dee-uul): Pertaining to after eating.

postpubertal (pohst-PYOO-ber-tuul): Occurring after sexual maturity.

pox (pahks): An eruptive or pustular disease, especially one caused by a virus.

practitioner (prak-TI-shuh-ner): One who is engaged in the diagnosis and treatment of diseases.

pre- (pree): Prefix meaning before, in time or space.

preadult (PREE-uh-**DAHLT**): Before maturity or before the adult period of life.

premolar (pree-MOH-ler): Tooth located rostral to the molars and caudal to the canine tooth.

preoperative (pree-AH-per-uh-tiv): Occurring before surgery.

preprandial (pree-PRAN-dee-uul): Before eating.

prepubertal (pree-PYOO-ber-tuul): Before sexual maturity.

prerenal (pree-REE-nuul): Situated cranial to the kidney or occurring before circulation to the kidneys.

prescription (preh-SKRIP-shuhn): Written direction for preparation and administration of a drug.

primi- (PRI-mi): Prefix meaning first.

primigravid (PRI-mi-**GRA**-vid): Pregnant for the first time.

primiparous (pri-MI-puh-ruhs): Having given birth once.

pro- (proh): Prefix meaning before or in front of.

process (PRAH-sehs): A projection or prominence on a bone; series of events or steps leading to a specific result.

Key to Pronunciation
a=hat • ah=hot • air=hair • al=bell • ay=day • eh=step • ee-deed • er=hurt
eye=fly • i=bit • oh=boa • too=boot • or=for • ow=cow • oy=joy • th=thin
uh=pup • uu=pull • y=fly • yoo=use • zh=measure

prochondral (proh-KAHN-druul): Occurring before formation of cartilage.

proct/o (PRAHK-toh): Combining form for rectum.

prodromal (proh-DROH-muul): Occurring before or indicating the onset of a disease or condition.

proestrus (proh-EH-struhs): Period preceding estrus or heat.

prognosis, prognoses (pl) (prahg-NOH-sis, prahg-NOH-seez): Forecast of the probable outcome of a disease.

prolapse (PROH-laps): Protrusion, falling down or sinking of an organ or part of an organ. Often implies eversion of an organ through normal body opening.

prolymphocyte (proh-LIM-foh-syt): Developmental stage of the lymphocyte series of white blood cells.

pronation (proh-NAY-shuhn): The act of turning to the prone position or turning a limb or part so the palmar or plantar surface is facing down.

prone (prohn): Lying with the face down in ventral recumbency.

prophylaxis (PROH-fi-**LAK**-sis): Prevention of disease.

proprietary name (proh-PRY-eh-**TEH**-ree): Trade or brand name of a drug.

prostat/o (prah-STA-toh): Combining form for prostate gland.

prostate (PRAH-stayt): An accessory sex gland in male animals of some species that surrounds the urethra in the pelvic canal.

prostatitis (PRAH-stuh-**TY**-tuhs): Inflammation of the prostate gland.

proventricul/o (PROH-vehn-**TRI**-kyoo-loh): Combining form for the proventriculus of birds.

proventriculus (PROH-vehn-**TRI**-kyoo-luhs): The glandular stomach of birds.

proximal (PRAHK-si-muul): Closer to any point of reference, or nearer to the center of the body or a part relative to another body part, or a location on a part relative to another more distant location.

pruritus (proo-RY-tuhs): Itchiness.

pseud/o (SOO-doh): Combining form meaning false.

pseudocyesis (SOO-doh-sy-EE-sis): False pregnancy, in which the signs of pregnancy exist but no fetus is present.

psittacine (SI-tuh-seen): Pertaining to birds of the parrot family, such as parrots, budgerigars and macaws.

psych/o (SY-koh): Combining form relating to the mind.

phychiatrist (sy-KY-uh-trist): Physician specializing in psychiatry, or mental illness.

psychologist (sy-KAHL-oh-jist): Specialist dealing with mental processes, especially behavior.

psychology (sy-KAHL-oh-jee): Branch of science dealing with mental processes, especially behavior.

psychomotor (SY-koh-**MOH**-ter): Pertaining to brain activity resulting in movement.

ptosis (TOH-sis): Drooping of the upper eyelid, generally due to the failure of the third cranial nerve; prolapse of an entire organ or part of an organ.

pub/o (PYOO-boh): Combining form for the pubis.

puberty (PYOO-ber-tee): Time at which an animal achieves sexual maturity and can reproduce.

pubis (PYOO-bis): The most ventral bone of the pelvis located on the floor of the pelvic canal.

pulmo, pulmon/o (PUUL-moh, puul-MAH-noh): Combining forms for the lungs.

Key to Pronunciation
a=hat • ah=hot • air=hair • al=bell • ay=day • eh=step • ee-deed • er=hurt
eye=fly • i=bit • oh=boa • too=boot • or=for • ow=cow • oy=joy • th=thin
uh=pup • uu=pull • y=fly • yoo=use • zh=measure

purulent (PYOO-roo-lehnt): Consisting of or containing pus.

pus (puhs): Liquid product of inflammation comprised of white blood cells, cellular debris and other matter.

putrefaction (PYOO-treh-**FAK**-shuhn): Decomposition by body enzymes, with production of foul-smelling compounds.

pyel/o (PY-eh-loh): Combining form for pelvis of the kidney.

pyelolithotripsy (PY-eh-loh-**LI**-thoh-trip-see): The crushing of a stone or calculus in the pelvis of a kidney.

pyelonephritis (PY-eh-loh-neh-**FRY**-tis): Inflammation of the kidney and its pelvis.

pylor/o (py-LOR-oh): Combining form for pylorus.

pyloromyotomy (py-LOR-oh-my-**AH**-toh-mee): Incision through the longitudinal and circular muscles of the pylorus, but not through the mucosa.

pyloroplasty (py-**LOR**-oh-PLA-stee): Surgical repair of the pylorus, generally done to enlarge the internal diameter of a strictured pylorus.

pylorus (py-LOR-uhs): The distal opening of the stomach into the duodenum.

pyo- (PY-oh): Prefix relating to pus.

pyometra (PY-oh-**MEE**-truh): Accumulation of pus in the uterus.

pyometritis (PY-oh-mee-**TRY**-tis): Inflammation of the uterus, with the presence of pus.

pyorrhea (PY-oh-**REE**-uh): Discharge of pus.

pyothorax (PY-oh-**THOR**-aks): Accumulation of pus in the pleural cavity.

pyrexia (py-REHK-see-uh): Fever.

pyuria (py-YOO-ree-uh): Pus in the urine.

Q

quad-, quadri- (kwahd, KWAH-dri): Prefix meaning 4.

quadrant (KWAH-druhnt): One-quarter of a circle, one section of a part or cavity arbitrarily divided into 4 areas.

quadriparous (kwah-DRI-puh-ruhs): Having had 4 pregnancies that resulted in viable offspring.

quadriplegia (KWAH-dri-**PLEE**-jee-uh): Paralyzed in all 4 limbs; tetraplegia.

quadruped (KWAH-droo-pehd): Animal with 4 feet.

queen (kween): Process of giving birth in cats; an adult intact female cat.

quick (kwik): The sensitive tissues of the claw or hoof.

R

radi/o (RAY-dee-oh): Combining form for the radius or radiation.

radiogram (RAY-dee-oh-gram): Image on film produced by pasage of x-rays through a body part.

radiograph (RAY-dee-oh-graf): A radiogram.

radiography (RAY-dee-**AH**-gruh-fee): The act or procedure of making a radiogram by use of an x-ray machine.

radiologist (RAY-dee-**AH**-loh-jist): Specialist in radiology.

radiology (RAY-dee-**AH**-loh-jee): Study of use of radiant energy (radiation) in diagnosis and treatment of disease.

radiolucent (RAY-dee-oh-**LOO**-sehnt): Permitting partial passage of radiation.

radiopaque (RAY-dee-oh-**PAYK**): Not permitting passage of radiation.

radiotransparent (RAY-dee-oh-tranz-**PEH**-rehnt): Permitting passage of radiation.

Key to Pronunciation

a=hat • ah=hot • air=hair • al=bell • ay=day • eh=step • ee-deed • er=hurt
eye=fly • i=bit • oh=boa • too=boot • or=for • ow=cow • oy=joy • th=thin
uh=pup • uu=pull • y=fly • yoo=use • zh=measure

radius (RAY-dee-uhs): The craniomedial bone of the foreleg between the elbow and carpal joint.

ramus (RAY-muhs): A branch; smaller structure that is part of a larger one.

re- (ree): Prefix meaning back, again, contrary, or replace.

recrudescence (REE-kroo-**DEH**-sehns): Recurrence of signs after temporary abatement.

rect/o (REHK-toh): Combining form for rectum.

rectocele (REHK-toh-seel): Herniation of part of the rectum into the vagina.

rectum (REHK-tuhm): The distal portion of the large intestine, ending at the anus.

recumbent (ree-KUHM-behnt): Lying down.

refracture (ree-FRAK-cher): To break a previously broken bone that was healed abnormally.

regurgitate (ree-GER-ji-tayt): To eject ingested food, specifically from the esophagus, when the food has not reached the stomach.

rehydrate (ree-HY-drayt): To replace lost body fluids.

relapse (ree-LAPS, REE-laps): Return of disease after apparent cure; recrudescence.

remission (ree-MI-shuhn): Diminution, lessening or abatement of signs of a disease; the period when signs of disease have abated or decreased.

ren/o (REE-noh): Combining form for kidney.

renopathy (ree-NAH-puh-thee): Any disease of the kidney; nephropathy.

resection (ree-SEHK-shuhn): Surgical removal or excision of a portion or of an entire organ or structure.

resident (REH-zi-dehnt): Graduate veterinarian or physician being trained in a specialty area in a hospital.

resistance (ree-ZI-stehns): Natural ability of the body to remain unaffected by poisonous substances and pathogenic microorganisms. In microbiology, it refers to lack of efficacy of a drug on a microorganism.

resorb (ree-ZORB): To take up or absorb again.

respiration (REH-spi-**RAY**-shuhn): The act of breathing; exchange of gases, such as oxygen and carbon dioxide, between the blood and body cells.

restraint (ree-STRAYNT): Forcible confinement by means of manually holding an animal or a body part to prevent movement during examination or treatment.

reticul/o (reh-TI-kyoo-loh): Combining form for reticulum.

reticulum (reh-TI-kyoo-luhm): The honeycombed second division of the stomach of ruminants.

retin/o (REH-ti-noh): Combining form for retina.

retina (REH-ti-nuh): The innermost layer of the eye, containing the cells that respond to light.

retro- (REH-troh): Prefix meaning backward or behind.

retrobulbar (REH-troh-**BAHL**-bahr): Behind the eyeball.

retroflexion (REH-troh-**FLEHK**-shuhn): Bending of an organ.

retroperitoneal (REH-troh-PAIR-i-toh-**NEE**-uul): Behind the peritoneum or between the peritoneum and body wall.

rheumatism (ROO-muh-tizm): Condition characterized by inflammation or degeneration of joints.

rhexis, -rrhexis (REHK-sis): Word or suffix meaning rupture.

rhin/o (RY-noh): Combining form for nose.

Key to Pronunciation

a=hat • ah=hot • air=hair • al=bell • ay=day • eh=step • ee-deed • er=hurt
eye=fly • i=bit • oh=boa • too=boot • or=for • ow=cow • oy=joy • th=thin
uh=pup • uu=pull • y=fly • yoo=use • zh=measure

rhinitis (ry-NY-tis): Inflammation of the mucous membranes of the nasal passages.

rhinoplasty (**RY**-noh-PLA-stee): Surgical reconstruction of the nose.

rhinorrhagia (RY-noh-**RA**-jee-uh): Nosebleed; epistaxis.

rigor mortis (RI-ger-**MOR**-tis): Stiffening of a dead body.

rostral (RAH-struul): Toward the nose (or beak), or pertaining to the nose end of the head or body.

rotation (roh-TAY-shuhn): Process of turning around an axis.

-rrhage, -rrhagia (raj, RA-jee-uh, RA-zhee-uh): Suffix meaning to burst forth or flow.

-rrhaphy (RUH-fee): Suffix meaning to suture together or join in a seam, a form of repair.

-rrhea (REE-uh): Suffix meaning flow or discharge.

rumen (ROO-mehn): Most proximal and largest division of the stomach in ruminants.

rumen/o, rumin/o (ROO-meh-noh): Combining forms for rumen.

rumenocentesis (ROO-meh-noh-sehn-**TEE**-sis): Withdrawal of fluid from the rumen using a needle inserted through the body wall.

rumenoectasia (ROO-meh-noh-ehk-**TAY**-zhee-uh): Dilatation of the rumen by accumulation of gas; bloat.

rumenostomy (ROO-meh-**NAH**-stoh-mee): Surgically created opening from the rumen to the body surface.

rump (ruhmp): Area around the point of the hips, tail, head and perineum.

S

sacr/o (SA-kroh, SAY-kroh): Combining form for sacrum.

sacrum (SAY-kruhm): Portion of the spinal column between the lumbar and coccygeal vertebrae, comprised of 3-5 fused vertebrae.

sagittal (SA-ji-tuul): A plane or line parallel to the median plane, separating the body or a part into right and left portions.

saline (SAY-leen, SAY-lyn): Salty; containing salts.

saliva (suh-LY-vuh): Clear, alkaline, viscid secretion from the mucous glands of the mouth.

salivary (SAL-i-veh-ree): Pertaining to saliva.

salping/o (sal-PIN-goh): Combining form relating to a tube, specifically the oviducts, or auditory tubes.

sanguineous (san-GWI-nee-uhs): Containing much blood.

saprophyte (SA-proh-fyt): Any organism living on dead tissue.

sarcoid (SAHR-koyd): Benign skin tumor of horses.

sarcoma, sarcomas or sarcomata (sahr-KOH-muh, sahr-KOH-muhs, sahr-KOH-muh-tuh): Malignant tumor derived from connective tissue cells.

saturated (SA-choo-RAY-tehd): Unable to hold in solution any more of a given substance; describing a fatty acid with all single bonds between carbon atoms.

scalpel (SKAL-puul): Small surgical knife with a straight handle and usually a detachable blade.

scapula (SKA-pyoo-luh): The flat, triangular bone that articulates with the humerus to form the shoulder joint; shoulder blade.

scapul/o (SKA-pyoo-loh): Combining form for scapula.

Key to Pronunciation
a=hat • ah=hot • air=hair • al=bell • ay=day • eh=step • ee-deed • er=hurt
eye=fly • i=bit • oh=boa • too=boot • or=for • ow=cow • oy=joy • th=thin
uh=pup • uu=pull • y=fly • yoo=use • zh=measure

scler/o (SKLEH-roh): Combining form for sclera; also prefix meaning hard or hardening.

sclera (SKLEH-ruh): The tough, white, outer tunic of the eyeball.

sclerosis (skleh-ROH-sis): Hardening of tissue, especially following inflammation.

scoliosis (SKOH-lee-**OH**-sis): Lateral deviation of the spine.

scope, -scope (skohp): A word or suffix meaning an instrument used for examining, viewing, listening or detecting.

-scopy (SKAH-pee, SKOH-pee): Suffix meaning the act of examining with an instrument.

scours (SKOW-erz): Common name for diarrhea in livestock.

scrot/o (SKROH-toh): Combining form for scrotum.

scrotum (SKROH-tuhm): The pouch containing the testes and their accessory organs.

scruff (skruhf): Common name for the loose skin around the neck and shoulders of dogs, cats and other small animals.

sedative (SEH-duh-tiv): Agent that reduces activity or decreases excitement.

seizure (SEE-zher): Sudden attack of a disease, especially neurologic disease; a convulsion.

semen (SEE-mehn): The thick, whitish reproductive secretion of males.

semi- (SEH-mee, SEH-my): Prefix meaning half or partially.

semiflexion (SEH-mee-**FLEHK**-shuhn): Position of the limb in partial flexion, or halfway between completely flexed and extended.

semipermeable (SEH-mee-**PER**-mee-uh-buul): Allowing the passage of certain molecules but hindering passage of others.

semiprone (SEH-mee-**PROHN**): Partially prone.

senile (SEE-nyl): Pertaining to old age.

sepsis (SEHP-sis): Presence of microorganisms or their toxins in the blood.

septicemia (SEHP-ti-**SEE**-mee-uh): Presence of microorganisms or their toxins in the blood.

septum, septa (pl) (SEHP-tuhm, SEHP-tuh): Dividing wall or partition.

serologic (SEH-roh-**LAH**-jik): Pertaining to antigen-antibody reactions.

serosa (seh-ROH-suh): Membrane lining a body cavity or investing an organ.

serous (SEH-ruhs): Pertaining to or resembling serum.

serum, sera (pl) (SEH-ruhm, SEH-ruh): The liquid portion of the blood remaining after removal of the clot and blood cells; the clear portion of a bodily liquid after removal of solid elements.

sesamoid bone (SEH-suh-moyd bohn): Small, nodular bone embedded between tendon and bone.

shoat (shoht): An immature weaned pig.

shock (shahk): Acute circulatory failure characterized by hypotension, cool extremities and rapid heart rate.

shunt (shuhnt): To divert or bypass; an abnormal connection between 2 natural vessels.

sial/o (SY-uh-loh): Combining form for saliva and salivary glands.

sigmoid (SIG-moyd): S-shaped.

sign (syn): Objective evidence of disease as perceived by the examining veterinarian.

sinus (SY-nuhs): Cavity or hollow space; abnormal channel formed for the escape of pus.

Key to Pronunciation
a=hat • ah=hot • air=hair • al=bell • ay=day • eh=step • ee-deed • er=hurt
eye=fly • i=bit • oh=boa • too=boot • or=for • ow=cow • oy=joy • th=thin
uh=pup • uu=pull • y=fly • yoo=use • zh=measure

sinus/o (SY-nuh-soh): Combining form for sinus.

sinusitis (SY-nuh-**SY**-tis): Inflammation of a paranasal sinus.

slough (sluhf): Dead tissue in the process of separating from adjacent viable tissue; to cast off or shed.

snout (snowt): The elongated nasal area of certain species, extending from the eyes rostrally to the nares.

solar (SOH-ler): Pertaining to the sun or the undersurface of a front foot.

sole (sohl): The undersurface of a front foot.

soma, soma-, -soma, somato- (SOH-muh, soh-MA-toh): Pertaining to the body or a body.

spasm, -spasm (SPA-zuhm): A sudden, violent, involuntary contraction of a muscle or group of muscles, generally accompanied by pain and impaired function; a sudden, brief, transitory constriction of a passage or orifice.

spavin (SPA-vin): A bony growth in the tarsal area of horses.

spay (spay): Ovariohysterectomy; to remove the ovaries and uterus of an animal.

specialist (SPEH-shuul-ist): Practitioner who concentrates on a particular branch of medicine or surgery.

specialty (SPEH-shuul-tee): Any particular branch of medicine.

species (SPEE-sheez, SPEE-seez): Category in classification of organisms, written in italics and following the genus name.

spectrum (SPEK-truhm): In pharmacology, the range of microorganisms against which a particular drug is effective.

speculum, specula (pl) (SPEHK-yoo-luhm), SPEHK-yoo-luh): Instrument used to expose a passage or body cavity.

spermatozoon, spermatozoa (pl) (sper-MA-toh-**ZOH**-ahn): The mature male germ cell.

sphincter (SFINK-ter): Ring-like band of muscle that closes a natural body opening.

sphygmomanometer (SFIG-moh-ma-**NAH**-meh-ter): Instrument used to measure arterial blood pressure.

spinal (SPY-nuul): Pertaining to the vertebral column.

spirometry (spy-RAH-meh-tree): Procedure of measuring the breathing capacity of the lungs.

splanchn/o (SPLANK-noh): Combining form for the viscera or the splanchnic nerve.

splanchnolith (SPLANK-noh-lith): An intestinal calculus or concretion; an enterolith or bezoar.

spleen (spleen): A large, oblong, reddish-purple, ductless gland, attached on the left side of the stomach or rumen, that stores red blood cells.

splen/o (SPLEH-noh): Combining form for spleen.

splenectomy (spleh-NEHK-toh-mee): Excision of the spleen.

splenomegaly (SPLEH-noh-**MEH**-guh-lee): Enlargement of the spleen.

splint (splint): A rigid or flexible appliance used to stabilize or prevent movement of a part; the second and fourth metacarpal and metatarsal bones in horses.

spondyl/o (SPAHN-di-loh): Combining form for the vertebral column.

spondylosis (SPAHN-di-**LOH**-sis): Fusion or ankylosis of a vertebral joint.

sprain (sprayn): Injury, but not rupture, of ligaments supporting a joint.

staphylo- (STA-fi-loh): Prefix denoting resemblance to a bunch of grapes.

Key to Pronunciation
a=hat • ah=hot • air=hair • al=bell • ay=day • eh=step • ee-deed • er=hurt
eye=fly • i=bit • oh=boa • too=boot • or=for • ow=cow • oy=joy • th=thin
uh=pup • uu=pull • y=fly • yoo=use • zh=measure

staphylococcus (STA-fi-loh-**KAH**-kuhs): A spherical bacterium that occurs in masses resembling a bunch of grapes; bacterium of the genus *Staphylococcus*.

stasis, -stasis (STAY-sis): Cessation of or reduced flow.

status (STA-tuhs): State or condition.

steer (steer): A castrated male bovine.

stenosis (steh-NOH-sis): Abnormal narrowing of a duct, vessel or tubular organ.

sterile (STEH-ril): Free of microorganisms; unable to reproduce.

stern/o (STER-noh): Combining form for sternum.

sternum (STER-nuhm): The ventral bone of the thorax, connecting all of the ribs ventrally.

steroid (STEH-royd): Compound in a group of chemicals, resembling cholesterol, that includes the sex hormones, glucocorticoids, mineralocorticoids and bile acids.

steroidal (steh-ROY-duul): Pertaining to steroids.

steth/o (STEH-thoh): Combining form relating to the chest.

stethoscope (STEH-thoh-skohp): Instrument used to listen to body sounds.

stifle (STY-fuul): The femorotibial joint; the "knee" of the rear leg.

stitch (stitch): Common term for a strand of material placed in tissue or skin with a needle to hold wound edges together for healing; a suture.

stoma (STOH-muh): An orifice or opening on a free surface; surgically created opening between anastomosed viscera.

stomach (STUH-mehk): The expanded part of the alimentary canal between the distal end of the esophagus and the proximal duodenum.

stomat/o (stoh-MA-toh): Combining form for mouth.

stomatoplasty (stoh-**MA**-toh-PLAS-tee): Surgery to repair a defect in the mouth.

-stomy (STOH-mee): Suffix relating to a surgically created opening into a hollow organ from the exterior surface of the body or an opening created by anastomosis of 2 hollow organs.

stool (stool): Feces.

stratum, strata (STRA-tuhm, STRA-tuh): One of several layers.

streak (streek): To distribute a microbiologic sample onto a plate of culture medium, usually with a swab or loop.

strepto- (STREHP-toh): Prefix meaning twisted.

streptobacillus, streptobacilli (pl) (STREHP-toh-buh-**SI**-luhs, STREHP-toh-buh-**SI**-ly): A rod-shaped bacterium occurring in twisted chains of bacteria linked end to end; bacteria of the genus *Streptobacillus*.

streptococcus, streptococci (pl) (STREHP-toh-**KAH**-kuhs, STREHP-toh-**KAH**-ky): A spherical bacterium occurring in linear groups resembling twisted chains; bacteria of the genus *Streptococcus*.

stricture (STRIK-cher): Area of reduced diameter in a passage or tubular organ as a result of scarring.

strip (strip): To manually remove milk from the udder.

stupor (STOO-per): Partial unconsciousness.

styptic (STIP-tik): An astringent or hemostatic agent.

sub- (suhb): Prefix meaning under, near, almost or moderately.

subacute (SUHB-uh-**KYOOT**): Of moderately rapid onset, between acute and chronic.

Key to Pronunciation

a=hat • ah=hot • air=hair • al=bell • ay=day • eh=step • ee=deed • er=hurt
eye=fly • i=bit • oh=boa • too=boot • or=for • ow=cow • oy=joy • th=thin
uh=pup • uu=pull • y=fly • yoo=use • zh=measure

subcutaneous (SUHB-kyoo-**TAY**-nee-uhs): Beneath the skin.

subluxation (SUHB-luhk-**SAY**-shuhn): Incomplete or partial dislocation.

subnormal (suhb-NOR-muul): Less than normal; below normal.

super- (SOO-per): Prefix meaning above or excess.

superficial (SOO-per-**FI**-shuul): Near the surface.

supernatant (SOO-per-**NAY**-tant): Overlying liquid after centrifugation or precipitation of solid.

supernumerary (SOO-per-**NOO**-mer-**AIR**-ee): Extra; in excess of the normal number.

supination (SOO-pi-**NAY**-shuhn): The act of turning to the supine position, or turning the limb so that the palmar or plantar surface is up.

supine (SOO-pyn): Lying face up, in dorsal recumbency.

suppository (suh-**PAH**-zi-**TOH**-ree): A medicated mass inserted into a body orifice, such as the rectum or vagina.

supra- (SOO-pruh): Prefix meaning above or over.

supranasal (SOO-pruh-**NAY**-zuul): Above the nose.

surgeon (SER-juhn): A doctor who performs surgeries.

surgery (SER-jeh-ree): A branch of medicine that treats disease by operative procedures; an operation; the place where operations are performed.

susceptible (suh-SEHP-ti-buul): Not immune to the actions of a pathogenic organism or an antimicrobial drug.

suture (SOO-cher): Material used to close a wound or tie off a bleeding vessel; type of fibrous union of tissue in which the opposed surfaces are closely united.

swage (swayj): Fusing of suture material to an eyeless needle.

sweeny (SWEE-nee): Common name for atrophy of the supraspinatus muscle in horses.

symptom (SIMP-tuhm): Subjective evidence of disease as perceived by a human patient.

syn- (sin): Prefix meaning together, in union or in association.

synalgia (sin-AL-jee-uh): Pain occurring in one location as a result of a lesion or problem in another location.

syndactyly (sin-DAK-ti-lee): Webbing or fusion of adjacent toes.

syndesm/o (sin-DEHZ-moh): Combining form for ligament or connective tissue.

syndrome (SIN-drohm): A set of clinical signs occurring together as the usual course of a disease or condition.

synergistic (SI-ner-**JIS**-tik): Acting together with enhanced effect.

synophthalmia (SIN-ahf-**THAL**-mee-uh): Fusion of both eyes into a single.

synostosis (SIN-ah-**STOH**-sis): Union of adjacent bones or parts of a single bone by ossification.

synovi/o (si-NOH-vee-oh): Combining form for synovium, joint fluid or joint capsule.

synovium (si-NOH-vee-uhm): The membrane lining a synovial joint and producing synovial fluid, a viscid fluid that lubricates the joint.

syringe, syringes (pl) (seh-RINJ, seh-RIN-jehz): Calibrated tubular instrument used for injecting or withdrawing liquids into or from the body.

syrinx, syringes (pl) (SEE-rinks, seh-RIN-jehz): Tube or pipe; the caudal larynx of a bird, where the voice is produced.

systemic (si-STEH-mik): Affecting the body as a whole.

Key to Pronunciation
a=hat • ah=hot • air=hair • al=bell • ay=day • eh=step • ee-deed • er=hurt
eye=fly • i=bit • oh=boa • too=boot • or=for • ow=cow • oy=joy • th=thin
uh=pup • uu=pull • y=fly • yoo=use • zh=measure

systolic (si-STAH-lik): Pertaining to the period when the heart ventricles are contracted to eject blood.

T

tachy- (TA-kee): Prefix meaning rapid.

tachycardia (TA-kee-**KAHR**-dee-uh): Excessively fast heart rate.

tachypnea (tuh-KIP-nee-uh): Excessively rapid respiration.

tamponade (TAM-poh-**NAHD**): Abnormal compression of the heart from accumulation of fluid in the sac surrounding the heart (pericardial sac).

tap (tap): To drain off fluid from a body cavity or fluid-filled sac by paracentesis.

tars/o (TAHR-soh): Combining form for tarsus.

tarsus (TAHR-suhs): The area distal to the tibia and fibula and proximal to the metatarsal bones.

tendon (TEHN-duhn): A fibrous cord by which muscle is attached to bone or to other muscles.

ten/o, tend/o, tendin/o (TEH-noh, TEHN-doh, TEHN-dinoh): Combining forms for tendon.

tenorrhaphy (teh-NOH-ruh-fee): Suturing a severed tendon.

tenosynovitis (TEH-noh-SI-noh-**VY**-tis): Inflammation of the sheath surrounding a tendon.

tension (TEHN-shuhn): The act of stretching, or being stretched or strained. Also used as a suffix related to the straining and stretching effect caused by pressure.

teratogenic (tair-A-toh-**JEH**-nik): Tending to produce birth defects.

terminology (TER-mi-**NAH**-loh-jee): Study of the system of scientific, medical or technical words and their component elements.

testicle (TEH-sti-kuul): Testis; the male gonad.

testicul/o (teh-STIK-yoo-loh): Combining form for testicle or testis.

testiculoma (teh-STIK-yoo-**LOH**-muh): A tumor originating from testicular tissue.

testis, testes (pl) (TEH-stis, TEH-steez): The male gonad, located in the scrotum in mammals, that produces spermatozoa and male hormones.

tetanus (TEH-tuh-nuhs): Infectious disease caused by the toxin produced by the bacterium *Clostridium tetani*, characterized by tonic muscular spasms; lockjaw.

tetra- (TEH-truh): Combining form meaning 4.

tetraplegia (TEH-truh-**PLEE**-jee-uh): Paralysis of all 4 extremities; quadriplegia.

therapeutic (THAIR-uh-**PYOO**-tik): Pertaining to treatment or healing.

therapy (THAIR-uh-pee): Treatment of disease.

theriogenologist (THAIR-ee-oh-jeh-**NAH**-loh-jist): Specialist in animal reproduction.

theriogenology (THAIR-ee-oh-jeh-**NAH**-loh-jee): Study of reproduction in animals.

therm/o (THER-mo): Prefix relating to heat.

thermophilic (THER-moh-**PHIL**-ik): Growing best at or having a fondness for high temperatures.

-thermia, -thermy (THER-mee-uh, THER-mee): Suffixes relating to heat.

thermic (THER-mik): Pertaining to heat.

thermogram (THER-moh-gram): Graphic record of the variation in body or environmental temperature.

Key to Pronunciation

a=hat • ah=hot • air=hair • al=bell • ay=day • eh=step • ee-deed • er=hurt
eye=fly • i=bit • oh=boa • too=boot • or=for • ow=cow • oy=joy • th=thin
uh=pup • uu=pull • y=fly • yoo=use • zh=measure

thermometer (ther-MAH-meh-ter): Instrument for measuring temperature.

thigh (thy): Area of the rear leg between the hip and the stifle.

thorac/o (THOR-oh-koh): Combining form for thorax.

thoracic (thor-A-sik): Pertaining to the thorax.

thorax (THOR-aks): The chest; section of the body between the neck and diaphragm.

thromb/o (THRAHM-boh): Prefix relating to a clot.

thrombolysis (thrahm-BAH-li-sis): Dissolution of a clot.

thrombus, thrombi (pl) (THRAHM-buhs, THRAHM-by): A blood clot. Also refers to a clot in a blood vessel that completely or partially obstructs the flow of blood, and remains at the site of origin.

throttle (THRAH-tuul): Common name for the throat or the ventral neck, including the larynx and trachea.

thrush (thruhsh): Common name for footrot or infection of the sole of the hoof in horses.

thyr/o (THY-roh): Combining form for thyroid gland.

thyroid (THY-royd): Paired gland, located on either side of the trachea, that produces hormones regulating body metabolism.

thyroidectomy (THY-roy-**DEHK**-toh-mee): Surgical removal of the thyroid gland.

tibi/o (TI-bee-oh): Combining form for tibia.

tibia (TI-bee-uh): The bone between the stifle and the tarsus, located medial to the fibula; the shin bone.

tic (tik): An involuntary, repetitive muscular contraction, usually of facial or shoulder muscles.

tissue (TI-shoo): An aggregation of cells specialized in one function.

toc/o (TOH-koh): Prefix related to the process of giving birth.

tocology (toh-KAH-loh-jee): Study of parturition; obstetrics.

tom (tahm): An intact adult male cat or turkey.

-tome (tohm): Suffix referring to an instrument used for cutting, or to a segment.

-tomy (TOH-mee): Suffix meaning to cut into or make an incision.

tonic (TAH-nik): Characterized by continuous tension or state of contraction.

tonometer (toh-NAH-meh-ter): Instrument used for measuring tension or pressure, specifically intraocular pressure in the eye.

tonsil (TAHN-sil): A small, rounded mass of lymphoid tissue, located bilaterally on either side of the dorsal part of the mouth just caudal to the glossopalatine arch.

tonsill/o (TAHN-si-loh): Combining form for tonsils.

tonsillectomy (TAHN-si-**LEHK**-toh-mee): Excision of one or both tonsils.

tonsillitis (TAHN-si-**LY**-tis): Inflammation of the tonsils.

topical (TAH-pi-kuul): Pertaining to a surface area.

torsion (TOR-zhuhn): Twisting or rotation.

tourniquet (TOR-ni-keht): Any device applied to an extremity or part to reduce blood flow.

tox/o, toxi-, toxic/o (TAHK-soh, TAHK-si, TAHK-si-koh): Prefixes relating to poisons.

toxemia (tahk-SEE-mee-uh): Condition resulting from bacterial toxins in the bloodstream.

toxicologist (TAHK-si-**KAH**-loh-jist): Specialist in poisons.

toxicology (TAHK-si-**KAH**-loh-jee): Study of poisons.

Key to Pronunciation

a=hat • ah=hot • air=hair • al=bell • ay=day • eh=step • ee-deed • er=hurt
eye=fly • i=bit • oh=boa • too=boot • or=for • ow=cow • oy=joy • th=thin
uh=pup • uu=pull • y=fly • yoo=use • zh=measure

toxicosis (TAHK-si-**KOH**-sis): Any condition caused by poisoning.

toxin (TAHK-sin): A poison.

toxoid (TAHK-soyd): A vaccine made of modified bacterial toxins, used to stimulate an immune response against toxins produced by those bacteria.

thrache/o (TRAY-kee-oh): Combining form for trachea.

trachea (TRAY-kee-uh): Tubular airway connecting the larynx to the bronchi.

tracheopathy (TRAY-kee-**AH**-puh-thee): Any disease of the trachea.

tracheotomy (TRAY-kee-**AH**-toh-mee): Incision into the trachea.

tranquilizer (**TRAN**-kwi-**LY**-zer): Drug used to calm an animal or relieve anxiety without necessarily altering consciousness or clarity of thought.

trans- (tranz): Prefix meaning across, through or beyond.

transfusion (tranz-FYOO-zhuhn): Introduction of whole blood or blood components into the bloodstream.

transient (TRAN-zhehnt): Temporary; passing away with time.

translucent (tranz-LOO-sehnt): Transmitting light, but diffusing it so that the objects behind it are not clearly visible.

transplantar (tranz-PLAN-ter): Across the sole of a rear hoof or foot.

transverse (trans-VERS): Placed crosswise, at a right angle to the long axis of a part or median plane of the body.

trauma, trauma-, traumat/o (TRAH-muh, trah-MA-toh): A wound or injury. The suffix relates to a wound or injury.

traumatic (trah-MA-tik): Pertaining to or as a result of injury.

traumatology (TRAH-muh-**TAH**-loh-jee): Study of injuries caused by trauma.

trephine (TREE-fyn): Special saw used to remove a circular core of bone.

tri- (try): Prefix meaning 3, triple or triplicate.

trich/o (TRY-koh): Combining form for hair.

trichobezoar (TRY-koh-**BEE**-zor): Concretion or solid mass of hair found in the stomach or intestine; a hairball.

trichophytobezoar (TRY-koh-FY-toh-**BEE**-zor): Concretion or solid mass of hair and vegetable matter found in the stomach or intestine.

tricuspid (try-KUH-spid): Having 3 points or cusps.

trilobectomy (TRY-loh-**BEHK**-toh-mee): Surgical removal of 3 lung lobes.

trimester (try-MEH-ster): A period of 3 months.

-tripsy (TRIP-see): The act of crushing.

trocar (TROH-kahr): Special large-bore needle used to puncture a body cavity for fluid withdrawal.

-trophic, -trophy (TROH-fik, TROH-fee): Suffix referring to tissue development based on nourishment of the constituent cells.

-tropic (TROH-pik): Suffix meaning turning toward or changing.

tubercle (TOO-ber-kuul): A small eminence on a bone; a small, rounded nodule produced by *Mycobacterium tuberculosis*.

tumescence (too-MEH-sehns): A swelling.

tumor (TOO-mer): A swelling or pathologic enlargement of tissues; a neoplasm.

turbid (TER-bid): Cloudy.

Key to Pronunciation
a=hat • ah=hot • air=hair • al=bell • ay=day • eh=step • ee-deed • er=hurt
eye=fly • i=bit • oh=boa • too=boot • or=for • ow=cow • oy=joy • th=thin
uh=pup • uu=pull • y=fly • yoo=use • zh=measure

twitch (twich): Device applied to the lip, ear or another part of horses for restraint during minor procedures; a brief, involuntary contraction of a skeletal muscle.

tympan/o (tim-PA-noh): Combining form for the tympanum, middle ear and eardrum.

tympanic membrane (tim-PA-nik MEHM-brayn): The eardrum.

tympanum (tim-PA-nuhm): The middle ear cavity, located medial to the tympanic membrane.

typhl/o (TIF-loh): Combining form from cecum.

U

ulcer (AHL-ser): A local defect or excavation of the surface of an organ or tissue, caused by sloughing of dead tissue.

uln/o (AHL-noh): Combining form for ulna.

ulna (AHL-nuh): The bone located caudolateral to the radius, between the humerus and the carpus.

ultra (AHL-truh): Prefix meaning beyond or extreme.

ultrasonography (AHL-truh-soh-**NAH**-gruh-fee): Use of ultrasonic waves to diagnose disease and delineate body structures by recording the resultant echoes.

-um (uhm): Suffix used to convert a positional or directional term to a noun meaning that aspect or area of the body designated by the root of the term to which it is attached.

umbilicus (uhm-BIL-i-kuhs): The navel; the scar marking the site of the fetal umbilical cord.

un- (uhn): Prefix meaning not, opposite of, reversal of, removal or release from.

uni- (YOO-ni): Meaning one or single.

unicellular (YOO-ni-**SAL**-yoo-ler): One-celled, or pertaining to a single-celled organism.

unilateral (YOO-ni-**LA**-teh-ruul): Affecting only one side.

unsaturated (uhn-**SA**-choo-**RAY**-tehd): Able to retain in solution more of a given substance; describing a fatty acid with one or more double or triple bonds between carbon atoms.

unsoundness (uhn-SOWND-nehs): In horses, any disease, condition or defect that causes lameness or an abnormal gait.

ur/o (YOO-roh): Combining form relating to urine, urination or the urinary system.

uremia (yoo-REE-mee-uh): Toxic condition, characterized by vomiting, anorexia, lethargy, neurologic signs, resulting from accumulation of nitrogenous urinary waste in the blood.

ureter (yoo-REE-ter): The fibromuscular tube that conveys urine from each kidney to the bladder.

ureter/o (yoo-REE-teh-roh): Combining form for ureter.

ureteropyosis (yoo-REE-teh-roh-py-**OH**-sis): Pus in the ureters, generally accompanied by inflammation.

urethr/o (yoo-REE-throh): Combining form for urethra.

urethra (yoo-REE-thruh): The tube that conveys urine from the bladder to the exterior of the body.

urethralgia (YOO-ree-**THRAL**-jee-uh): Pain in the urethra.

urethrorrhagia (yoo-REE-throh-**RA**-jee-uh): Hemorrhage or flow of blood from the urethra.

urethrostomy (YOO-ree-**THRAH**-stoh-mee): Surgical creation of a permanent opening in the urethra in the perineum or another area.

-uria (YOO-ree-uh): Suffix referring to a characteristic or constituent of urine.

urin/o (YOO-ri-noh): Combining form relating to urine.

urinalysis (YOO-ri-**NAL**-i-sis): Analysis of urine by chemical and microscopic examination.

Key to Pronunciation

a=hat • ah=hot • air=hair • al=bell • ay=day • eh=step • ee-deed • er=hurt
eye=fly • i=bit • oh=boa • too=boot • or=for • ow=cow • oy=joy • th=thin
uh=pup • uu=pull • y=fly • yoo=use • zh=measure

urination (YOO-ri-**NAY**-shuhn): Passage or discharge of urine.

urine (YOO-rin): Fluid formed in the kidneys, passed to the bladder for storage, and discharged through the urethra.

urogenital (YOO-roh-**JEH**-ni-tuul): Pertaining to urinary and genital structures.

urolith (YOO-roh-lith): Stone or calculus in the urinary system.

urolithiasis (YOO-roh-li-**THY**-uh-sis): Condition character-ized by calculi in the urinary system.

urologist (yoo-**RAH**-loh-jist): Specialist in diseases of the uri-nary system.

urology (yoo-**RAH**-loh-jee): Study of disorders of the urinary system.

urticaria (ER-ti-**KAIR**-ee-uh): Raised, red patches of skin, often accompanied by itchiness; hives.

uter/o (YOO-teh-roh): Combining form for uterus.

uteropexy (**YOO**-teh-roh-PEHK-see): Surgical fixation of the uterus to the body wall or another structure to prevent tor-sion or displacement; hysteropexy.

uterus (YOO-teh-ruhs): A hollow muscular organ, located in the caudal abdominal cavity of female mammals, in which the fertilized ovum develops.

uve/o (YOO-vee-oh): Combining form for uvea.

uvea (YOO-vee-uh): The vascular middle layer of the eye, con-sisting of the iris, ciliary body and choroid.

V

vaccine (VAK-seen): A suspension of killed or attenuated mi-croorganisms that, when introduced into the body, stimulates an immune response against that microorganism.

vagin/o (VA-ji-noh): Combining form for vagina.

vagina (vuh-JY-nuh): The canal in females, extending from the vulva to the cervix, that receives the penis during copulation.

valgus (VAL-guhs): Angled away from the midline of the body.

varus (VEH-ruhs): Angled toward the midline of the body.

vas/o (VA-zoh, VAY-zoh): Combining form relating to vessels or ducts.

vasoconstriction (VA-zoh-kahn-**STRIK**-shuhn): Decrease in the diameter of a blood vessel, especially an arteriole.

vasodilation (VA-zoh-dy-**LAY**-shuhn): Increase in the diameter of a blood vessel, especially an arteriole.

vehicle (VEE-hi-kuul): Any medium through which an impulse may be passed; an inert substance with which a drug is mixed before administration.

vein (vayn): Vessel through which blood returns from organs and body parts to the heart.

ven/o (VEE-noh, VEH-noh): Combining form for vein.

venipuncture (**VEH**-ni-**PUHNK**-cher): Puncture of a vein with a needle.

ventilation (VEHN-ti-**LAY**-shuhn): The process of exchanging air between the lungs and the atmosphere; the process of replacement of air in a room or building by mechanical means.

ventral (VEHN-truul): Pertaining to the belly or underside of the quadruped, or denoting a position more toward the belly (downward) than some other reference point or body part.

ventricle (VEHN-tri-kuul): A small cavity, such as the cavities of the brain or the lower chambers of the heart.

ventricul/o (vehn-TRI-kyoo-loh): Combining form for a ventricle of the brain or heart.

ventro- (VEHN-troh): Combining form denoting a position more toward the belly than some other reference point.

venule (VEHN-yuul): Very small vessels that collect blood from the capillaries, then join to form veins.

vertebra, vertebrae (pl) (VER-teh-bruh, VER-teh-bray): The bones of the spinal column, divided into cervical, thoracic, lumbar, sacral and coccygeal vertebrae.

vertebrate (VER-teh-brayt): Any animal with a spinal column; having a spinal column.

vertebro (VER-teh-broh): Combining form for vertebrae.

vesic/o (VEH-si-koh): Combining form relating to the bladder or a blister.

vesicle (VEH-si-kuul): Small sac or blister containing fluid.

vessel (VEH-suul): Any channel, tube or duct for carrying fluid, such as blood or lymph.

veterinarian (VEH-teh-ri-**NAIR**-ee-uhn): Doctor of veterinary medicine.

veterinary (VEH-teh-ri-**NAIR**-ee): Pertaining to domestic animals and their diseases.

viable (VY-uh-buul): Capable of living; remaining alive.

viremia (vy-REE-mee-uh): Viruses in the blood.

virology (vy-RAH-loh-jee): Study of viruses and the diseases they produce.

virulence (VEER-yoo-lehns): The degree of pathogenicity of a microorganism; the degree to which a microorganism can cause serious disease.

virus (VY-ruhs): A minute infectious agent that replicates only inside a living cell, and lacks the ability for independent metabolism.

viscer/o (VI-seh-roh): Combining form for the viscera.

viscous (VIS-kuhs): Sticky or adhesive.

viscus, viscera (pl) (VIS-kuhs, VI-seh-ruh): Any large organ located within the thoracic or abdominal cavities, or within the pelvic canal.

vital (VY-tuul): Necessary for life.

vivi- (VI-vi): Combining form relating to life.

viviparous (vy-VI-puh-ruhs): Bearing live young, as in mammals.

volar (VOH-ler): Pertaining to the undersurface of the front feet or the caudal aspect of the front legs of quadrupeds.

volvulus (VAHL-vyoo-luhs): Twisting of the bowel to the point of causing obstruction.

vomit (VAH-mit): To cast up material from the stomach; the material cast up from the stomach.

vomitus (VAH-mi-tuhs): Material cast up from the stomach.

vulv/o (VAHL-voh): Combining form for vulva.

vulva (VAHL-vuh): External genitalia of females, including the labia and vaginal opening.

vulvovaginitis (VAHL-voh-VA-ji-NY-tis): Inflammation of the vulva and vagina.

W

wall (wahl): The horny, hard epidermal tissue comprising the outer surface of the hoof of livestock; the limiting tissue surrounding a cavity, such as the abdominal wall surrounding the abdominal cavity or the cell wall surrounding intracellular contents.

wattle (WAH-tuul): The fleshy outgrowth of skin about the beak of birds or hanging from the chin or throat of a goat or turkey.

Key to Pronunciation

a=hat • ah=hot • air=hair • al=bell • ay=day • eh=step • ee-deed • er=hurt
eye=fly • i=bit • oh=boa • too=boot • or=for • ow=cow • oy=joy • th=thin
uh=pup • uu=pull • y=fly • yoo=use • zh=measure

wean (ween): To discontinue nursing or suckling a young animal.

weanling (WEEN-ling): Young animal recently changed from suckling to another source of food.

wether (WEH-ther): A castrated male sheep.

whelp (wehlp): The process of giving birth in dogs; an unweaned puppy.

white line (wyt lyn): A pale line on the periphery of the sole of the hoof, adjacent to the hoof wall, representing the continuation of the insensitive laminae to the wall; common term for the linea alba, on the abdominal midline, dividing the rectus muscles.

withers (WI-therz): The top or highest point of the shoulders of horses.

Wood's light (wuudz lyt): An ultraviolet light, often used to detect fluorescent fungi on the skin of animals.

wound (woond): Any disruption of the continuity of a normal structure, as from incision or injury.

X

xanth/o (ZAN-thoh): Prefix meaning yellow.

xanthocyte (ZAN-thoh-syt): Cell containing yellow pigment.

xanthoma (zan-THOH-muh): Yellow plague, papule or nudule in the skin formed by lipid deposits.

xenograft (ZEE-noh-graft): Transplant or graft of tissue between different species; a heterograft; a heterotransplant.

xero (ZEE-roh): Combining form meaning dry.

xeroradiography (ZEE-roh-RAY-dee-**AH**-gruh-fee): A dry photoelectric process of making radiographic images.

xerostomia (ZEE-roh-**STOH**-mee-uh): Dryness of the mouth.

x-ray (EHKS-ray): An electromagnetic vibration used to diagnose and treat disease.

Z

zoo- (ZOH-oh): Combining form relating to animals.

zoologic medicine (ZOH-oh-**LAH**-jik MEH-di-sin): A branch of veterinary medicine dealing with diseases and husbandry of zoo animals and wild and exotic species.

zoonosis, zoonoses (pl) (ZOH-oh-**NOH**-sis, ZOH-oh-**NOH**-seez): A disease of animals that can be transmitted to people, under natural conditions.

Key to Pronunciation
a=hat • ah=hot • air=hair • al=bell • ay=day • eh=step • ee-deed • er=hurt
eye=fly • i=bit • oh=boa • too=boot • or=for • ow=cow • oy=joy • th=thin
uh=pup • uu=pull • y=fly • yoo=use • zh=measure

Appendix 3

Bibliography

Agnew LRC *et al: Dorland's Illustrated Dictionary*. 27th ed. Saunders, Philadelphia, 1988.

Blair JE *et al: Manual of Clinical Microbiology*. Williams & Wilkins, Baltimore, 1970.

Blood DC and Radostits OM: *Veterinary Medicine*. 7th ed. Saunders, Philadelphia, 1988.

Blood DC and Studdert VP: *Bailliere's Comprehensive Veterinary Dictionary*. Saunders, Philadelphia, 1989.

Borrow DJ: *Dictionary of Root Words and Combining Forms*. N-P Publications, Palo Alto, CA, 1971.

Catcott EJ: *Animal Health Technology*. American Veterinary Publications, Goleta, CA, 1977.

Complete Equipment & Supplies for the Veterinary Practice. Les Wilkins & Associates, Seattle.

Davis LE: *Handbook of Small Animal Therapeutics*. Churchill Livingstone, New York, 1985.

Elster CH: *There is No Zoo in Zoology*. Macmillan, New York, 1988.

Fenner F *et al: Veterinary Virology*. 3rd ed. Academic Press, San Diego, 1986.

Frandson RD: *Anatomy and Physiology of Farm Animals*. 4th ed. Lea & Febiger, Philadelphia, 1986.

Getty R: *Sisson and Grossman's The Anatomy of the Domestic Animals*. 5th ed. Saunders, Philadelphia, 1975.

Griffiths HJ: *A Handbook of Veterinary Parasitology, Domestic Animals of North America*. Univ Minnesota Press, Minneapolis, 1978.

Guralnik DB *et al: Webster's New World Dictionary of the American Language*. 2nd college ed. Simon & Schuster, New York, 1984.

Handy-Marchello B: *The Veterinary Technician's Guide to Medical Terminology*. Reston Publishing, Reston, VA, 1984.

Hensyl WR: *Stedman's Pocket Medical Dictionary*. Williams & Wilkins, Baltimore, 1987.

Holmes DD: *Clinical Laboratory Animal Medicine*. Iowa State Univ Press, Ames, 1984.

Jackson JC: *New American Pocket Medical Dictionary*. Longman, New York, 1978.

Leach M *et al: Functional Anatomy, Mammalian and Comparative*. McGraw-Hill, New York.

McCurnin DM: *Clinical Textbook for Veterinary Technicians*. 2nd ed. Saunders, Philadelphia, 1990.

Evans HE and Christenson GC: *Miller's Anatomy of the Dog*. 2nd ed. Saunders, Philadelphia, 1979.

Misdom-Frank Instrument Catalog. Misdom-Frank Instrument Co, West Chester, PA, 1983.

Prendergast A: *Medical Terminology: A Text/Workbook*. 2nd ed. Addison-Wesley Publishing, Menlo Park, CA, 1983.

Picker GD: *Dosage Calculations*. 2nd ed. Delmar Publications, Albany, NY, 1987.

Wroble EM: *Terminology for the Health Professions*. Lippincott, Philadelphia, 1982.